Dr.Jesus

# Dr. Jesus

## Devotions for Your Mental Health

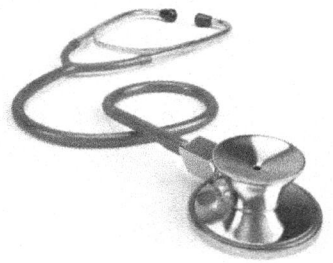

Michael Caparrelli, Jr., PhD

Copyright © 2021 by Michael A. Caparrelli.
All rights reserved. This book or any portion thereof
may not be reproduced or used in any manner whatsoever
without the express written permission of the publisher
except for the use of brief quotations in a book review.

Published by UNMUTED Publications

Visit: unmuted.app
Contact: unmuted777@gmail.com

Back Cover Photo: Rebecca Daniele
(Facebook: Radiance by Rebecca Photography)
Interior & Cover Design: Sarah Vaas

Unless otherwise stated, scripture quotations are NIV
from The Holy Bible, New International Version® NIV®
Copyright © 1973 1978 1984 2011 by Biblica, Inc.
Used by permission. All rights reserved worldwide.

Scripture quotations from the ESVr Bible
(The Holy Bible, English Standard Version®), copyright © 2001
by Crossway Bibles, a publishing ministry of
Good News Publishers. Used by permission. All rights reserved.

# CONTENTS

FOREWORD ...................................................................................................... 1
INTRODUCTION .............................................................................................. 3
ADDICTION: ..................................................................................................... 7
ATTENTION DEFICIT DISORDER (A.D.D.): ............................................. 19
ANTI-SOCIAL: ................................................................................................ 27
ANXIETY: ........................................................................................................ 35
BIPOLAR: ........................................................................................................ 41
BORDERLINE PERSONALITY DISORDER: ............................................. 47
CODEPENDENCY: ......................................................................................... 53
CRISIS: ............................................................................................................. 59
DEPRESSION: ................................................................................................. 65
EATING DISORDER: ..................................................................................... 81
FATIGUE: ........................................................................................................ 85
GENERATIONAL CURSE: ............................................................................ 93
GRIEF: .............................................................................................................. 99
HOARDING: .................................................................................................. 107
INSECURITY: ................................................................................................ 113
NARCISSISM: ............................................................................................... 123
OBSESSIVE COMPULSIVE DISORDER: .................................................. 129
PARANOIA: ................................................................................................... 133
POST-TRAUMATIC STRESS DISORDER: ................................................ 139
RELATIONSHIP STRIFE: ............................................................................ 147
STRESS: ......................................................................................................... 159

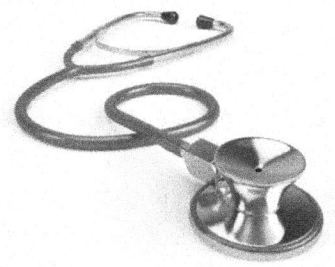

# FOREWORD

I am honored to present this book to you. Dr. Mike Caparrelli is a friend of many years. I've watched his life, example, and ministry. Every conversation I have with him results in my life being better, my ministry being enriched, and my soul being encouraged. You can experience the same thing as you work through this set of devotional readings.

What happens when someone is deeply challenged with mental illness? Then, they find their way out of it as a direct result of their faith in God. Next, they become a pastor and plant a church. In that context, they offer a place of healing and hope for those who struggle with mental illness. Finally, they devote years of study to obtain a PhD in Behavioral Science. Mix all of that journey together and you have this collection of devotionals found in this book.

As Christ followers, we have many voices addressing the topics of mental illness, addiction, depression etc. What Mike brings is a life story, a pastoral journey and academic rigor. All these experiences are deposited into each of these devotionals.

Mike opens up his own journey in very real, raw and tangible ways. He lays a Biblical framework for each devotional. This approach allows his story to come alongside the Biblical narrative and leads us to reflect on our lives. Then, to brilliantly dig deeper, he provides a path of reflection questions at the end of each devotional. These questions are the invitation to an understanding and a path forward.

As you read through these devotionals, you will find great hope for yourself and those you care for. Whether you are a ministry leader, small group leader or journeying on your own path to freedom and wholeness, these devotionals are a gift. Ministry leader, this book on your shelf will be a tool to navigate situations with those who are struggling with their mental health. Small group leader, here is a track for your group to run on toward a life of freedom and joy. For you, there are devotionals here that every human on the planet will find helpful.

While it is not prescriptive, it is surely pastoral. Mike is careful not to hand out a solution; rather, he offers you a path to the God who cares, sets free and gives peace. As Mike would say, we need to meet Dr. Jesus. If you pick this up as a reference for a specific situation in your life or a friend, you will have a robust resource; one that is funny, readable and powerful all at the same time. This unique approach is an accessible help for the wide-ranging challenges of mental health we all face at different levels and different seasons. No doubt, reading it occasionally or regularly will help you and those you care for.

Thank you, Dr. Cap, for this practical gift.  - Nick Fatato

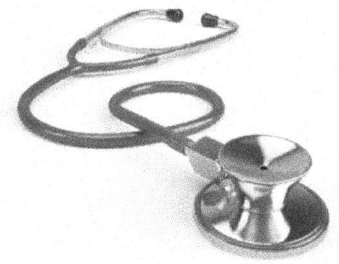

# INTRODUCTION

Let me say something about Meds. "Paxil, Lithium and Klonopin ensure that I will never fall into another funk again". That's what I presumed at 15 years old when my shrink wrote me scripts for these drugs at copious dosages after years of reckless euphoria followed up by long-lasting melancholiac spells. These drugs were the Messiah I sought for! Conversely, reality bit me in the wazoo. I figured out there were no egresses from the heartache of being dumped by your girlfriend, the anxiety associated with school exams or the inner turmoil that ensues family strife. Funks were a part of human existence that called for a level of maturity to navigate through without plunging too deep. Yes, the meds dulled the edge of the blade called mental illness, but I still needed to develop the E.Q. required for surviving in this world. Pills don't teach skills.

Let me say something about Institutions. "Butler Psychiatric Hospital is a great resort for mental health holidays". That's how I reasoned throughout my adolescence every time I felt like bolting from the ordeals of life. Of course, Butler Hospital kept me alive on several occasions. But, after countless mental health holidays, institutions morphed from being a reality into becoming a mentality. I soon became institutionalized whereby my strength to function within the real world under duties, demands and deadlines was sapped. When a man knows he's got a place to hide, he's less likely to square off with the giants before him. Institutions enabled me to pull a Houdini (disappearing act) whenever life got too hard.

Let me say something about Psychologists. Truthfully, I haven't had many good shrinks through the years. At the risk of being cynical, I've come to the grim conclusion that my mental maladies equated to their job security. If I ever got well, God forbid, my wholeness meant they were one step closer to being unemployed. During therapy sessions, I felt like I was type-casted by the shrink into playing a whack-job for the rest of my life. Like a child star that couldn't get away from the stigma of early television roles, I felt incapable of landing any normal parts. Psychologists, at least for me, were accomplices to my insanity.

Let me say something about the System. At 18 years old, after years of hospitalizations, I applied for Social Security Income (SSI). Strangely enough, I was approved the first time for $700 per month, free medical insurance, food stamps and a handful of other freebies. All of the system's financial benefits served to my detriment. How? The hopes of ever getting better were far removed from my mind given the fact that I didn't want to lose the perks that came with being sick. I understood clearly why Jesus asked the lame man in John 5, "Do you want to get well?", – getting better meant losing his livelihood! He made a living off his handicap by begging people for money for 38 years. Being free from his handicap was tantamount to being unemployed. Unregulated benevolent systems often make slaves out of otherwise able bodies.

Meds, shrinks, nut houses and systems, for me, were no antidotes. Undoubtedly, each of these natural means aided my survival during the earlier years of my life. I would never recommend anyone to cut ties with prescriptions, psychologists or psych wards in view of the fact that these might be the only lifelines they have. But, for me, these resources were only temporary reprieves from a deep-seated insanity.

In November 1996, just a few days after my 18th birthday, I encountered Dr. Jesus during a church service in Rhode Island after Pastor Pasco Manzo preached a sermon from the gospel of John. No doubt, the psychological healing in my life from that moment forward didn't happen suddenly but subtly. Nonetheless, a cataclysmic shift occurred on that evening that set me free from the grip of mental illness. It just took time for my mind to grasp what happened in my spirit all at once. Twenty-six years later, the evidence speaks for itself – I live a reasonably happy life, married with seven children, hold a PhD in Behavioral Science, authored several books and teach at a local college...all without taking any prescription meds, receiving Social Security Income or mental health holidays at local psych hospitals. A good shrink, on the other hand, who also knows Dr. Jesus, is an invaluable part of my healing journey.

Of course, I still get into funks. A funk is a natural response to being betrayed by loved ones, disappointed by the world or losing something precious. Whoever expects life to be devoid of heartaches and headaches is searching for something that cannot be had on this side of heaven. So, there are funks. But, as the scripture pledges, these funks "come to pass" rather than coming to stay. During these times, I partake the spiritual meds prescribed to me within His Word. Dr. Jesus' counsel, along with the guidance of His Physician Assistants (the apostles who penned the bible under divine inspiration), is *"Spirit and Life"* (John 6:63). *Spirit* means He gives me the power to be whom He crafted me to be, and *Life* means He gives me the eyes to see the existence He predestined for me to see.

Throughout this devotional, you will discover daily commentaries on the biblical verses that played a pivotal role in my healing. These daily meditations were (and still are) my daily medication. Take note that Dr. Jesus' counsel, along with the words of His assistants, is wholistic, remedying every dimension of our makeup – physical, mental, emotional, social, existential and spiritual. Furthermore, each daily commentary features scientific research from the scholars of behavioral science that confirms Dr. Jesus' counsel.

My prayer is that whatever heartaches you have – depression, anxiety, post-traumatic stress, etc. – will be remedied through these meditations. You will see, that long before the emergence of Freud, Jung, Erickson or Bandura, Dr. Jesus made His house calls. He shows to be the final expert on human behavior. You don't just read His words, but His words read you. As you peruse the pages of this book, please allow the great doctor to mend your fractured soul. Be of good cheer, there is a doctor in the house!

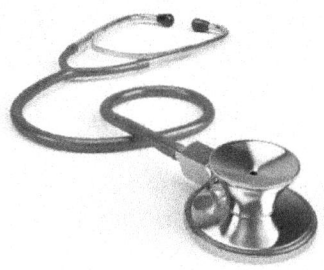

# ADDICTION:

*A chronic relapsing pattern characterized by compulsive, stimuli-seeking behaviors despite the consequences ensued.*

RELEVANT BIBLICAL PERSONALITIES:
The Prodigal Son (Luke 15:11-13)
Lemuel (Proverbs 31:1-7)
Solomon (I Kings 11:1-8)
Noah (Genesis 9:21-23)
David (II Samuel 11:1-27)

## M.Y.O.B. - A KEY TO DEFEATING ADDICTION

*Make it your ambition to lead a quiet life: you should mind your own business
and work with your hands. I Thessalonians 4*

Improper passing occurs when you cross over into someone else's lane without a proper opening. Being a belligerent driver in a bygone era, I had my share of traffic violations, verbal altercations, and even collisions from improper passes. Similarly, most clashes within relationships happen with improper passing, such as when you stick your nose into a situation without any right of entry. The Apostle teaches us what life in the Spirit looks like – he basically says, "M.Y.O.B. - Mind Your Own Business." Staying in your own lane ensures a safer journey on many levels (of course, there's always the possibility of someone crossing into your lane, but that warrants an entirely different devotional).

How does this relate to addiction? Cortisol, a stress hormone, escalates when we take on a role higher than our aptitude. If you've ever seen the anxiety of a rookie managing the store after the supervisor calls in sick, you've witnessed how assuming other people's jobs causes stress. Likewise, you'll find yourself frazzled when you manage other people's lives, such as interjecting with your grown kid's situations, interfering with your neighbor's dilemmas, or getting too wrapped up in politics. The weight of research shows that cortisol spikes constitute a significant risk factor of relapse with illicit substances (Sinha, 2008). Take heed –such stress is not a far cry from a sip, a snort, or any slip.

"Work with your hands", the Apostle states shortly after warning us to mind our own business. The statement alludes to Adam and Eve, who tilled the garden with their hands before dialoguing with the serpent. Under the spell of the serpent, Eve became distracted with the affairs of God ("You shall become like god") while neglecting the work of her hands. The Apostle is telling us, go back to what Adam and Eve were doing before they fell from grace. Maintaining sobriety means managing YOUR world instead of trying to govern THE world. Once again, staying in your lane proves to be the safest way of navigating through this wild terrain.

### Related Verses:
*Ecclesiastes 2:24, Colossians 3:23-24, II Thessalonians 3:11-12*

DR. JESUS

# DAILY M.E.D.S.:

*Apply this tool to receive the medicinal benefits of the devotional from the previous page.*

## MEDITATE:
Reflect upon the content of this devotional. Write, recite and mull over the key verses repeatedly until they reach your heart.

_____
_____
_____
_____

## ENGAGE:
Discuss this devotional with a trusted spiritual friend, pastor or counselor. Share your struggles relating to this devotional. Write whatever significant feedback they offer you. Most importantly, incorporate this devotional into your prayer life.

_____
_____
_____
_____

## DECIDE:
Consider the practical decisions you must make regarding this devotional. Write down those decisions and seek someone to keep you accountable.

_____
_____
_____
_____

## SURVEY:
Take note of your progress regarding this devotional. Changes don't happen suddenly but subtly. Write down any subtle improvements you notice over some time.

_____
_____
_____
_____

# OVERCOMING BOREDOM:
## A Key in Defeating Addiction
*"Idle hands are the devil's workshop; idle lips his mouthpiece." Proverbs 16:27*

Monotony can be more uncomfortable than agony. A team of psychologists at the University of Virginia ascertained that 2/3rds of men and 1/4th of women prefer self-administered shocks over being left alone in a room for 15 minutes with nothing to do (Wilson, 2014). For this reason, folks will do just about anything to escape the humdrum life. Regarding addiction, boredom is a top risk factor of reckless behaviors such as substance abuse. On the darker side, F.B.I. agents discovered a prevalent theme of "a hollow existence, a profound boredom" within their in-depth interviews with mass murders about their lives before the atrocities. Satan scouts the human population for blasé recruits with no meaningful pursuits to carry out his dirty deeds. I venture to say that most people who relapse were twiddling their thumbs in boredom, just a few minutes before the devil's knock.

Monotony often results from a disconnect between your tenets and your tasks. Your tenets are what you hold within your heart, whereas tasks are what you hold within your hands. When your hearts and your hands don't link up, monotony is the outcome. If you can't see the significance behind sweeping the floor or tucking the kids in at night, hollowness fills your mind. In Hebrew, the term idle is defined as "worthless" and "good for nothing." As stated before, when your deeds are devoid of meaning, you place a welcome mat outside your temple for the devil and his cohorts.

A little review - First, you overcome addictions partly by reducing boredom (a.k.a monotony). Second, you curtail boredom by linking your tenets with your tasks. With that said, conduct an audit today on what you believe. Please take heed, if you can't link your tenets with your tasks, Satan will eventually bait you into his business. To quote G.K. Chesterson, "The problem with a lack of belief in God is not that it leads to a belief in nothing, but that it leads to belief in anything." The idle mind is, in fact, the devil's workshop.

---

### Related Verses:
*Proverbs 13:4, Philippians 4:8, Ecclesiastes 9:10*

# DAILY M.E.D.S.:

*Apply this tool to receive the medicinal benefits of the devotional from the previous page.*

### MEDITATE:
Reflect upon the content of this devotional. Write, recite and mull over the key verses repeatedly until they reach your heart.

_____
_____
_____
_____

### ENGAGE:
Discuss this devotional with a trusted spiritual friend, pastor or counselor. Share your struggles relating to this devotional. Write whatever significant feedback they offer you. Most importantly, incorporate this devotional into your prayer life.

_____
_____
_____
_____

### DECIDE:
Consider the practical decisions you must make regarding this devotional. Write down those decisions and seek someone to keep you accountable.

_____
_____
_____
_____

### SURVEY:
Take note of your progress regarding this devotional. Changes don't happen suddenly but subtly. Write down any subtle improvements you notice over some time.

_____
_____
_____
_____

# HEALING A WOUNDED SELF-IMAGE:
## A Key to Defeating Addiction

*"It is not for kings, O Lemuel, it is not for kings to drink wine; nor is strong drink for princes."* Proverbs 31:4

A KING resides within every man. The KING signifies the noble part of you that rationally governs your impulses while influencing the world around you for the better. The KING is cool. Alongside the KING, there is also a KID. The KID reflects the out-of-control child with reckless appetites, the bad-boy who pays a high price for a low life. The KID is a fool. Addiction happens when you hand the keys over to the KID while putting the KING to sleep. In Proverbs 31:4, a wise mother helps her addicted son, Lemuel, by awakening the KING from his coma to take control of the KID. Lemuel is a drunkard partly because he's forgotten who he is. Thank God for a mom who reminds him of his royal pedigree.

Behavioral scientists show through innumerable studies that self-image plays a pivotal role in recovery from substances. For instance, in a study performed at London South Bank University amongst 61 people attending A.A. meetings (2013), researchers found that relapse rates were significantly higher amongst those who identified as "addicts" versus "recovering addicts". Of course, some will say that eliminating the term "addict", altogether provides better results. Either way, self-image shows to be critical in sobriety. Your chances of a successful recovery skyrocket when you awaken to who you are – a KING destined for greatness, and not just some reckless K.I.D.

Ladies, the same principle applies to you. Historians tell us that Queen Victoria was once a rascal who upset the royal family with her shenanigans. One day, her teacher informed her that she was in line for the throne, a destiny that her family cloaked from her eyes. With this knowledge at hand, little Victoria arose from being a scoundrel to becoming a woman of noble character. Suddenly, she had no time for foolish games. God created you in his Royal likeness; leave the silly games for kids.

---

### Related Verses:
*Genesis 1:26-27, Psalm 139:14, Colossians 3:10*

# DAILY M.E.D.S.:

*Apply this tool to receive the medicinal benefits of the devotional from the previous page.*

## MEDITATE:
Reflect upon the content of this devotional. Write, recite and mull over the key verses repeatedly until they reach your heart.

_____
_____
_____
_____

## ENGAGE:
Discuss this devotional with a trusted spiritual friend, pastor or counselor. Share your struggles relating to this devotional. Write whatever significant feedback they offer you. Most importantly, incorporate this devotional into your prayer life.

_____
_____
_____
_____

## DECIDE:
Consider the practical decisions you must make regarding this devotional. Write down those decisions and seek someone to keep you accountable.

_____
_____
_____
_____

## SURVEY:
Take note of your progress regarding this devotional. Changes don't happen suddenly but subtly. Write down any subtle improvements you notice over some time.

_____
_____
_____
_____

# BREAKING BAD HABITS

*"Anyone who steals should steal no more but do something useful w/ his hands."*
*Ephesians 4:28*

How do you know you're enslaved to something? When you inhale cheesecake despite your passionate plan to lose 20lbs, you have a problem. You spent an hour ranting to your sister about your ever-expanding waistline. Seconds later, you're placing your order with Grub-Hub for that graham-cracker-crusted delicacy. Yesteryear, you nibbled on cheesecake merely because it was pleasurable. Well, that era is long gone! Now you eat cheesecake because it's irresistible. When the pleasurable evolves into the irresistible, your neurology has been twisted into a double fisherman knot. Slavery is NOT when you do something because you get to do it (that's voluntary service). Rather, slavery is when you do something because you got to do it. You have lost all autonomy.

Now, let's ask the essential question – how do you break bad habits? This question lends itself to endless strategies but let's focus on just one. Miller et al. (1960) established that breaking bad habits begins with pursuing another goal that somehow corresponds to the bad habit but offers greater satisfaction. The Apostle Paul's instruction for thieves (those addicted to stealing) to work with their hands is an excellent example of Miller et al.'s theory in practice. The itch to shoplift disappears when you get busy with your hands and subsequently enjoy the fruit of your labor. In an era without neuroscience, the Apostle Paul, under the unction of the Spirit knew that breaking bad habits starts with forming alternative habits. A new love is the best cure for recovering from an old dangerous love.

On a personal note, I know I'm addicted to criticizing customer service because I just can't stop! Standing in line at the grocery store yesterday, I quickly noticed the reason for the long wait – the young cashier was sipping on her Caramel Frapuccino in between scanning items. It'd be indecent to repeat some of my raging thoughts. A gloating smile sprinted across my face when she dropped her Frappuccino all over the floor. "That'll teach her!". As I was leaving the mart, it felt like my addiction to nitpicking was just reinforced by that spill. Suddenly, I heard God say, "Go buy her another Frappuccino." God was saying to me, "Do you want to kick your addiction to criticizing? Then, show appreciation". Kicking and screaming, I brought that young cashier a new drink after waiting in another long, annoying line at Starbucks. I'm not virtue-signaling, believe me. I fully recognize I have a loooong way to go in this area. But, one of the surest ways of breaking old habits is forging new ones.

### Related Verses:
*I Corinthians 9:27, Galatians 6:8, Matthew 5:16*

# DAILY M.E.D.S.:

*Apply this tool to receive the medicinal benefits of the devotional from the previous page.*

## MEDITATE:
Reflect upon the content of this devotional. Write, recite and mull over the key verses repeatedly until they reach your heart.

_____
_____
_____
_____

## ENGAGE:
Discuss this devotional with a trusted spiritual friend, pastor or counselor. Share your struggles relating to this devotional. Write whatever significant feedback they offer you. Most importantly, incorporate this devotional into your prayer life.

_____
_____
_____
_____

## DECIDE:
Consider the practical decisions you must make regarding this devotional. Write down those decisions and seek someone to keep you accountable.

_____
_____
_____
_____

## SURVEY:
Take note of your progress regarding this devotional. Changes don't happen suddenly but subtly. Write down any subtle improvements you notice over some time.

_____
_____
_____
_____

ADDICTION

## WHY BEING STILL IS SO GRUELING?
*"He makes me lie down in green pastures...He restores my soul." Psalm 23:2-3*

Being still is a grueling task for those who've escaped addiction. Every addict owns a pair of running shoes. It begins with running away from a chaotic home, resumes with running the streets and ends with running from the police. When your survival hinges on intensity, stillness feels dangerous, as if something awful is about to catch up with you. Taking off your running shoes to sit in the presence of God defies every survival instinct flaring within you.

From a neurological perspective, addicts are adrenaline junkies. Epinephrine, a.k.a. adrenaline, is a hormone released within your bloodstream when you're moving. A tremendous benefit of adrenaline is that it numbs your body from pain; hence, soldiers resume within war even after being shot several times. Adrenaline is a natural opiate that anesthetizes you from physical and emotional agony. The problem with being still is that adrenaline subsides, or the painkiller wears off. All your painful emotions bubble to the surface; the grief from losing your mother, the sting of rejection from the wife who left you, the resentment towards your father who abandoned you. What makes stillness so grueling is that you must face off with what you feel.

In Psalm 23:2, the Psalmist uses forceful language, "He makes me lie down...". Shepherds often apply a "leg break" to make sheep lie down. A leg brake is a cumbersome weight tied to the ankle of a wandering sheep to tire its body. What are the "leg brakes" God uses to make you still? Sickness, unemployment, a traffic jam? Know that in those moments of stillness, He's not trying to torture you but restore your soul. Face-off with what you feel, and allow the Good Shepherd to walk you through the valley of death.

---

### Related Verses:
*Psalm 46:10, I Kings 19:12, Psalm 23:4*

# DAILY M.E.D.S.:

*Apply this tool to receive the medicinal benefits of the devotional from the previous page.*

## MEDITATE:
Reflect upon the content of this devotional. Write, recite and mull over the key verses repeatedly until they reach your heart.

_____
_____
_____
_____

## ENGAGE:
Discuss this devotional with a trusted spiritual friend, pastor or counselor. Share your struggles relating to this devotional. Write whatever significant feedback they offer you. Most importantly, incorporate this devotional into your prayer life.

_____
_____
_____
_____

## DECIDE:
Consider the practical decisions you must make regarding this devotional. Write down those decisions and seek someone to keep you accountable.

_____
_____
_____
_____

## SURVEY:
Take note of your progress regarding this devotional. Changes don't happen suddenly but subtly. Write down any subtle improvements you notice over some time.

_____
_____
_____
_____

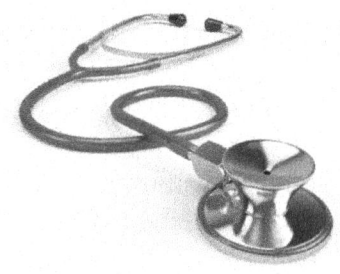

# ATTENTION DEFICIT DISORDER (A.D.D.):

*Habitual symptoms of inattentiveness, distractions, and a poor working memory.*

### RELEVANT BIBLICAL PERSONALITIES:
Martha (Luke 10:41)

Peter (Matthew 17:4, John 18:10)

Lame Man (Acts 3:4)

Esau (Genesis 25:29-24)

A.D.D.

# SELECTIVE ATTENTION SPAN
*"My Sheep Know My Voice." John 10:27*

Let's face it - in some cases, Attention Deficit Disorder (A.D.D.) is nothing more than a pathetic cover-up for a person's lack of prioritizing, valuing or investment in something. The renowned cocktail-party experiment (Cherry, 1953) revealed that participants were incapable of hearing the conversations of their peers at a cocktail party...that is, UNTIL their names were mentioned. Suddenly, their ears perked up like the antenna of a 1990's cell phone. The cocktail party experiment made it loud and clear that homo-sapiens pay close attention to data relevant to their self-interests. Let me break it down for you this way....

Once upon a time, a Catholic monk and a business tycoon strolled through Central Park, Manhattan. "Take note to the robin's song, the howling of the wind, the rustling of the waterfall," the monk whispered to the tycoon. "I'm sorry, brother, but I can't hear much of what you mentioned. My hearing is bad", the tycoon replied. After a few minutes passed, the monk deliberately dropped a quarter on the pavement. After hearing the sound of the coin's drop, the tycoon bent down to pick it up. The monk glanced at him and said, "Bad hearing, 'eh? Whatever captures your affection holds your attention".

In John 10:27, Jesus employs the personal pronoun, 'My', to describe his followers – "My sheep". The term refers to His gentle hold upon their hearts. His usage of 'My' is much like a woman tenderly saying about her lover, "My man". Jesus is saying with the term My, "I have their hearts". Now, notice the second half of the verse – "know my voice". Here, Jesus describes his follower's ability to distinguish His voice amidst all other noises. Jesus is saying, "I have their ears." In summary, Jesus says, "Because I hold their hearts, I have their ears." If you struggle with paying attention to something or someone, perhaps the issue lies within your heart. You instinctively pay attention to whatever holds your affections. Set your affections on the right things, and those right things will hold your attention.

---

**Related Verses:**
*Proverbs 1:33, Colossians 3:2, James 1:19*

# DAILY M.E.D.S.:
*Apply this tool to receive the medicinal benefits of the devotional from the previous page.*

### MEDITATE:
Reflect upon the content of this devotional. Write, recite and mull over the key verses repeatedly until they reach your heart.

_____
_____
_____
_____

### ENGAGE:
Discuss this devotional with a trusted spiritual friend, pastor or counselor. Share your struggles relating to this devotional. Write whatever significant feedback they offer you. Most importantly, incorporate this devotional into your prayer life.

_____
_____
_____
_____

### DECIDE:
Consider the practical decisions you must make regarding this devotional. Write down those decisions and seek someone to keep you accountable.

_____
_____
_____
_____

### SURVEY:
Take note of your progress regarding this devotional. Changes don't happen suddenly but subtly. Write down any subtle improvements you notice over some time.

_____
_____
_____
_____

A.D.D.

# IMPROVING YOUR FOCUS (PART 1)

*"On the Sabbath, we went outside the city gate to the river, where we expected to find a place of prayer. We sat down and began to speak to the women who had gathered there."*
Acts 16:13

Studies indicate that the average person can focus no longer than 90 minutes before requiring a break. Let's face it - some of us have the attention span of a mosquito at a picnic with no longer than a few seconds of concentration before shifting to something else. A sure way of improving your focus is dividing your task into intervals of time (10, 15 or 20-minute intervals) where you allow yourself even 45 seconds of mental retreat between each segment (Ariga & Lleras, 2011). Have you ever seen the movie "A Few Good Men"? You might remember Tom Cruise's character playing with his baseball bat while prepping for litigation. It turns out that the bat relaxes him enough to think sharply. The mind needs a balance of effort and ease to stay focused.

Undoubtedly, the Apostle Paul was a focused missionary who worked hard in Macedonia building up the local churches. But even the industrious Paul needs a break! In Acts 16:13, he leaves the city for prayer and fellowship on the Sabbath day. Understand that Sabbath, for the Jews, meant so much more than our American understanding of rest. We, Americans, define rest as mere relaxation. The Jews understood rest as restoration. When Paul leaves the city for prayer and fellowship, he's not just relaxing but restoring his mind's ability to focus.

Think of a violin. If the strings aren't sufficiently stretched, you'll produce a sound too dull to be in tune. But if the strings are stretched too much, you run the risk of snapping the four steel cords. For the violin to play sharply, the strings require a proper balance of tension and relaxation. In the same way, your mind is the sharpest when you give it just enough effort and ease. So, to improve your focus, make a cup of coffee, call your B.F.F. or swing a golf club during predetermined intermission breaks.

---

### Related Verses:
*Matthew 11:28-30, Hebrews 4:1-11, Isaiah 14:3-4*

# DAILY M.E.D.S.:

*Apply this tool to receive the medicinal benefits of the devotional from the previous page.*

## MEDITATE:
Reflect upon the content of this devotional. Write, recite and mull over the key verses repeatedly until they reach your heart.

_____
_____
_____
_____

## ENGAGE:
Discuss this devotional with a trusted spiritual friend, pastor or counselor. Share your struggles relating to this devotional. Write whatever significant feedback they offer you. Most importantly, incorporate this devotional into your prayer life.

_____
_____
_____
_____

## DECIDE:
Consider the practical decisions you must make regarding this devotional. Write down those decisions and seek someone to keep you accountable.

_____
_____
_____
_____

## SURVEY:
Take note of your progress regarding this devotional. Changes don't happen suddenly but subtly. Write down any subtle improvements you notice over some time.

_____
_____
_____
_____

# IMPROVING YOUR FOCUS (Part 2)
*"Seek first the kingdom of God and His righteousness, and all these things will be added to you." Matthew 6:33*

Being fully persuaded by your priorities is crucial in remaining focused. Haphazard goals leave you vulnerable to every distraction you stumble upon. Minutia, the petty details that randomly pop up throughout the performance of a task, hijack your attention quickly if you do not know what's most important. For instance, you casually decide to install a birdhouse in your backyard. Sure, you like birds, and birdhouses are fun, but it's one of those things you can live without. With this casual posture, you jump at your cell phone every time it hums. Edwin Locke, a psychologist who specialized in goal-setting, discovered that having clearly defined goals you wholeheartedly believe is the key to successful outcomes (Locke, 1996).

Dr. Jesus describes a person with a Midas touch in Matthew 6:33; in other words, the kind of man or woman who prospers in every endeavor. The phrase, "added to you" speaks of gain on every level – financial, social, intellectual, and spiritual gains. Such an individual engages in few, if any at all, boondoggles (projects that bear no fruit) in their life. In the first half of Matthew 6:33, Dr. Jesus sheds light on the key for such prosperous living – make the Kingdom of God "first". The term, 'first', means a priority that consumes you like an obsession you can't shake. The term, 'first', means something that has the utmost priority in your life. This kind of posture is the best insulation against petty distractions. Let me say it this way....

As soon as Milwaukee Braves power-hitter Hank Aaron stepped up to bat, opponent Yogi Berra heckled him incessantly. "Henry, you're holding the bat wrong! You're supposed to hold it the other way so you can read the trademark!". After Aaron knocked the ball out of the park and ran full circuit around the bases, he approached the dugout where Yogi hid. He said, "I didn't come here today to read trademarks." Aaron knew his priority; therefore, he wasn't distracted by petty things. Being fully convinced of your purpose is one of the best deterrents against the hecklers of life.

---

## Related Verses:
*Proverbs 4:25, Proverbs 16:33, Matthew 6:24*

# DAILY M.E.D.S.:

*Apply this tool to receive the medicinal benefits of the devotional from the previous page.*

## MEDITATE:
Reflect upon the content of this devotional. Write, recite and mull over the key verses repeatedly until they reach your heart.

_____
_____
_____
_____

## ENGAGE:
Discuss this devotional with a trusted spiritual friend, pastor or counselor. Share your struggles relating to this devotional. Write whatever significant feedback they offer you. Most importantly, incorporate this devotional into your prayer life.

_____
_____
_____
_____

## DECIDE:
Consider the practical decisions you must make regarding this devotional. Write down those decisions and seek someone to keep you accountable.

_____
_____
_____
_____

## SURVEY:
Take note of your progress regarding this devotional. Changes don't happen suddenly but subtly. Write down any subtle improvements you notice over some time.

_____
_____
_____
_____

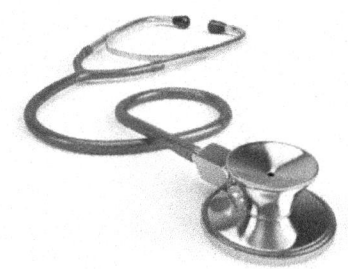

# ANTI-SOCIAL:

*Socially maladjusted behaviors that defy the norms, rules and laws of a community along with hostile, cold, and manipulative attitudes.*

### RELEVANT BIBLICAL PERSONALITIES:
Paul (Acts 8:1, I Timothy 1:13)

David (II Samuel 11:6-24)

Reprobates (Romans 1:20-28)

Herod (Matthew 2:16)

Samson (Judges 13-16)

# OBJECTIFICATION

*"She (Pharoah's daughter) opened it and saw the baby. He was crying, and she felt sorry for him. 'This is one of the Hebrew babies,' she said." Exodus 2:5-6*

Serial killers pull off heinous crimes against humanity by perceiving their prey as items rather than individuals. The notorious B.T.K. (Bind Torture Kill) identified his victims as "projects" rather than people. Similarly, pornography filmmakers showcase their seductive stars, not as whole people with genuine personalities, but fleshly parts - extreme close-ups of lips, hips and whatever else. All crimes against humanity (Violence, porn, or whatever else) require objectification, a cognitive process by which we diminish a soul into an object. Why? Because it's easy to abuse or misuse an inanimate article. It's rather painstaking to mistreat a living entity.

Yale University psychologist Stanley Milgram recruited participants to administer electrical shocks under a doctor's instructions to a particular subject in an experiment. Milgram performed the study to understand the psychology behind Nazi tormenters (1961). Unbeknownst to the participants, the shocks were fictitious, and the subjects were players in the experiment. Milgram learned, amongst many other discoveries, that there occurred a lesser likelihood of participants administering shocks if they held the subjects' hands. The study shows that close and personal exposure to people heightens our empathy, which subsequently lowers our possibility of cruelty. Empathy is the antidote to savagery.

In our passage of study, something magnificent happens to Pharoah's daughter. From a distance, Hebrew children were merely a statistic she read about in the latest edition of the Egyptian Times. From a distance, Hebrew tots were nothing more than one of the many babies her father annihilated; what the historians call, "The Massacre of the Hebrew Sons." From a distance, Pharoah's daughter's heart was probably indifferent towards such a massive genocide. But now, up close and personal, staring into the eyes of this helpless baby, objectification dissolves and compassion awakens! She sees the loveable baby and can't resist helping. All this to say, if you're running low on love, draw a little closer to the people whom you've given the cold shoulder. Distance chills the heart while proximity warms it up. Stalin hit the nail on the head when he stated, "The death of millions is a statistic, whereas the death of one is a tragedy."

---

### Related Verses:
*Matthew 24:12, II Timothy 3:2, Ezekiel 36:26*

# DAILY M.E.D.S.:

*Apply this tool to receive the medicinal benefits of the devotional from the previous page.*

### MEDITATE:
Reflect upon the content of this devotional. Write, recite and mull over the key verses repeatedly until they reach your heart.

_____
_____
_____
_____

### ENGAGE:
Discuss this devotional with a trusted spiritual friend, pastor or counselor. Share your struggles relating to this devotional. Write whatever significant feedback they offer you. Most importantly, incorporate this devotional into your prayer life.

_____
_____
_____
_____

### DECIDE:
Consider the practical decisions you must make regarding this devotional. Write down those decisions and seek someone to keep you accountable.

_____
_____
_____
_____

### SURVEY:
Take note of your progress regarding this devotional. Changes don't happen suddenly but subtly. Write down any subtle improvements you notice over some time.

_____
_____
_____
_____

ANTI-SOCIAL

# HOW BEING CLIQUEY IS COSTLY

*"Do not forget to show hospitality to strangers, for by so doing some people have shown hospitality to angels without knowing it." Hebrews 13:2*

Being cliquey is second nature for we homo sapiens. Cliques surface quickly within any community because of the law of propinquity. The law of propinquity states that friendships form easiest with the people physically closest to us. In a classic experiment of the 1950s, researchers established that 41% of residents claimed a close relationship with their neighbor one door away, 22% with the neighbor two doors away and 10% with neighbors down the hall of an apartment building (Festinger et al., 1950). Simply being in the proximity of someone increases the likelihood of a bond. Sir Peter Ustinov stated in his autobiography, 'Dear Me', "I do not believe that friends are the people you like the best; they are merely the people who got there first."

Take heed because cliquey is costly. Tight bonds often result in an "Us Four and No More" vibe that shuns all new kids on the block. While this exclusive mentality may feel comfortable, it's intellectually and emotionally consequential. Regarding intellectual consequences, you're bound to suffer from a parochial worldview (a limited perspective on life) by surrounding yourself with the same opinions day after day. Think of it this way, a picture colored with only one or two crayons is lackluster compared to a portrait with many crayons. Regarding emotional consequences, codependency is an easy trap for being with the same folks every day. Codependency is an inordinate reliance upon someone to meet certain needs.

The Greek term for hospitality in Hebrews 13:12 is Philo-Xenos, an oxymoronic word with rich meaning. Philo means "brotherly love" while Xenos means "the perfect stranger"; this composite word is defined as "Loving the perfect stranger as a beloved brother". Philo-Xenos (hospitality) is a challenge for those who fall prey to propinquity, gravitating towards neighbors while giving the cold shoulder to foreigners. But for those willing to step outside your comfort zone, you just might brush shoulders with an angel who holds the key to some promise. The Apostle Paul tells us, "By embracing strangers, you might be encountering angels." Divine visitations await those who welcome strangers.

---

### Related Verses:
*Isaiah 58:7, 1 Peter 4:8-9, Leviticus 19:33-34*

# DAILY M.E.D.S.:

*Apply this tool to receive the medicinal benefits of the devotional from the previous page.*

## MEDITATE:
Reflect upon the content of this devotional. Write, recite and mull over the key verses repeatedly until they reach your heart.

_____
_____
_____
_____

## ENGAGE:
Discuss this devotional with a trusted spiritual friend, pastor or counselor. Share your struggles relating to this devotional. Write whatever significant feedback they offer you. Most importantly, incorporate this devotional into your prayer life.

_____
_____
_____
_____

## DECIDE:
Consider the practical decisions you must make regarding this devotional. Write down those decisions and seek someone to keep you accountable.

_____
_____
_____
_____

## SURVEY:
Take note of your progress regarding this devotional. Changes don't happen suddenly but subtly. Write down any subtle improvements you notice over some time.

_____
_____
_____
_____

# AM I PREJUDICED?

*"As Peter entered, Cornelius met him and fell at his feet in reverence....Peter said, 'You are well aware that it is against our law for a Jew to associate with or visit a Gentile. But God has shown me that I should not call anyone impure.'" Acts 10:25, 28*

Categorizing people, places and things is a basic human instinct. Playing in the sandbox, you lined up your toy soldiers in fictitious squads according to size, color, or some other criteria. A few years later, you organized your school documents in a Trapper Keeper according to the subject. Because of your inherent need for order, you've been categorizing your entire life based on similarities.....But generalizing (aka prejudice) is not the same as categorizing. Categorizing is the ability to spot the similarity between things, whereas generalizing is the inability to notice the difference between things.

Out-Group Homogeneity is defined as perceiving outsiders as being all the same. The empirical evidence for this concept is astounding, most notably an experiment amongst 90 college students (Park, Rothbaft, 1982). Participants were asked by researchers to predict preferred music genres within their college as well as other colleges. Researchers found that participants judged their sorority members with a diverse range of music genres. In contrast, students from other colleges were considered to have the same taste. The experiment shows that we judge insiders rightly but judge outsiders stereotypically. For example, we might say, "Oh, he's just another liberal", "Oh, she's just another Trump supporter!". What's known as 'the law of least effort' inhibits us from getting to know people intimately, causing our perceptions to be painted over with a broad brush.

When Peter visits with the gentile named Cornelius, the kind of man he formerly shunned, he encounters someone who doesn't fit the stereotype. According to Peter, gentiles are as well-mannered as prehistoric savages. But that's not the case with Cornelius. He's courteous, reverent and generous, a slap against every stereotype Peter held about gentiles. This visit was equally for Peter's sake as it was for Cornelius' soul. To all the Peters of the world - not all Blacks play basketball, not all Italians have a kingpin godfather, not all cops are trigger happy racists, and not all gentiles are uncouth pagans. Resist your anti-social impulses, and you'll be pleasantly surprised by the people you once judged.

---

### Related Verses:
*I Corinthians 12:13, I John 2:11, I Samuel 16:7*

# DAILY M.E.D.S.:

*Apply this tool to receive the medicinal benefits of the devotional from the previous page.*

## MEDITATE:
Reflect upon the content of this devotional. Write, recite and mull over the key verses repeatedly until they reach your heart.

_____
_____
_____
_____

## ENGAGE:
Discuss this devotional with a trusted spiritual friend, pastor or counselor. Share your struggles relating to this devotional. Write whatever significant feedback they offer you. Most importantly, incorporate this devotional into your prayer life.

_____
_____
_____
_____

## DECIDE:
Consider the practical decisions you must make regarding this devotional. Write down those decisions and seek someone to keep you accountable.

_____
_____
_____
_____

## SURVEY:
Take note of your progress regarding this devotional. Changes don't happen suddenly but subtly. Write down any subtle improvements you notice over some time.

_____
_____
_____
_____

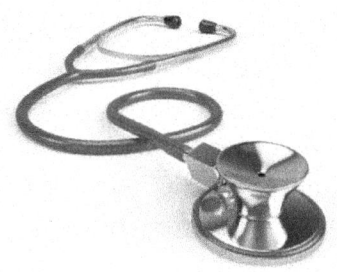

# ANXIETY:

*Feelings of tension, worried thoughts and physiological changes such as increase of blood pressure, dilated pupils, and tightened muscles.*

RELEVANT BIBLICAL PERSONALITIES:
Martha (Luke 10:40-42)
Job (Job 2:1, 11, 20-22, 26)
Jonah (Jonah 4:3)
Moses (Exodus 3:11, 4:13)
Children of Israel (Numbers 13:31-33)

# TREATING ANXIETY

*"And we know that in all things God works for the good of those who love him, who have been called according to His purpose." Romans 8:28*

I knew my mother already watched the suspenseful flick, "Silence of the Lambs," based on her body language. We agreed to view the rented Blockbuster VHS together when I returned home from high school, but she evidently beat me to the punch. How did I know she saw it already? As Dr. Hannibal Lector outwitted his jailors with barbaric methods, my mom wasn't nibbling her nails, toying with her hair, or pacing the floor. Her composure in the face of tension squealed on her. Being an intuitive kid with a probing glare, I said, "You watched the movie without me, huh?". She couldn't hide her smirk. Only a woman who already viewed the glorious ending was capable of coolness in the nerve-wracking middle. Mom had a sense of certainty of how the movie would end, therefore, was less stressed during suspenseful scenes. Anxiety always subsides where certainty resides.

Conversely, according to a study from the University of Illinois at Chicago, uncertainty is at the root of various neurotic psychopathologies (Gorka et al., 2016). An experiment amongst 160 participants revealed significantly more anxious eye-blinks (motorized by your cerebellum) amongst individuals subjected to unpredictable electrical shocks compared to folks subjected to shocks that followed a clockwork pattern. In darker research, many parents of missing children admit to feeling solace when investigators notified them of finding their child's corpse. How so? Known facts subdued the unknown possibilities within their minds. Whether you're waiting for that dreaded phone call from the doctor or that nauseating meeting with your employer, uncertainty is what's fueling your anxiety.

Romans 8:28 dramatically reduces the suspense of everyday existence for those of us who live and love in God. Romans 8:28 works stronger than Benzos by promising that all agony will culminate into ecstasy as God works everything out into a glorious conclusion. Romans 8:28 gives us a glimpse of our final destination. "And we know that...." is not speculative guesswork but a sure conviction that this is how it will all end! We who've read the end of the Good Book can rest serenely in the middle of our stories.

---

## Related Verses:
*Proverbs 3:5-6, Colossians 3:23-24, Jeremiah 29:11*

# DAILY M.E.D.S.:

*Apply this tool to receive the medicinal benefits of the devotional from the previous page.*

## MEDITATE:
Reflect upon the content of this devotional. Write, recite and mull over the key verses repeatedly until they reach your heart.

_____
_____
_____
_____

## ENGAGE:
Discuss this devotional with a trusted spiritual friend, pastor or counselor. Share your struggles relating to this devotional. Write whatever significant feedback they offer you. Most importantly, incorporate this devotional into your prayer life.

_____
_____
_____
_____

## DECIDE:
Consider the practical decisions you must make regarding this devotional. Write down those decisions and seek someone to keep you accountable.

_____
_____
_____
_____

## SURVEY:
Take note of your progress regarding this devotional. Changes don't happen suddenly but subtly. Write down any subtle improvements you notice over some time.

_____
_____
_____
_____

## IS GRATITUDE MORE POTENT THAN ANXIETY?

*"Be anxious for nothing, but in everything by prayer and supplication, with THANKSGIVING, let your requests be made known to God." Philippians 4:6*

It is common knowledge amongst academics that gratitude produces manifold psychological benefits. The real question is, "Does gratitude produce these same benefits amongst those with clinical conditions such as anxiety disorder?" Researchers endeavored to examine the effects of gratitude-writing amongst 300 college students with a clinical diagnosis. Gratitude-writing was defined as penning letters that expressed appreciation to benefactors (family, friends, etc). Researchers found that gratitude-writing not only reduced anxiety levels amongst participants within the four weeks of the study but even at a post-study 12-week follow-up point (Wong et al., 2016). The investigation revealed that gratitude is more sturdy than anxiety.

From a neuroscience perspective, here's how gratitude triumphs over anxiety. Additional fMRI scans indicate that gratitude activates the medial prefrontal cortex, the part of the brain that solves problems. How does this relate to anxiety? Anxiety flourishes within the minds of people who hyper-focus on problems rather than solutions. Anxious people are those who rehearse and rehash what's wrong without ever considering how to fix it. Gratitude shifts the brain from problem-focused thinking to solution-oriented cognition. Through the lens of gratitude, anxiety lowers as we perceive giants as defeat-able rather than unbeatable.

Note something significant about the gratitude (thanksgiving) that the Apostle Paul pits up against anxiety in Philippians 4. It is not merely gratitude that is thankful FOR something, but gratitude that is thankful TO someone. The phrase, "...to God", says it all. Even in the gratitude-writing study mentioned above, participants expressed their thankfulness, not just FOR something, but TO someone. Today, summon to mind all of the people you should give thanks TO; most notably, express your gratitude to the Savior who gave His life for you. Resultant of this exercise, you will notice that worries fall at the wayside. You will understand why the Apostle Paul encourages anxious people to be thankful.

**Related Verses:**
*Ezra 3:11, James 1:17, Luke 17:11-19*

Dr. JESUS

# DAILY M.E.D.S.:
*Apply this tool to receive the medicinal benefits of the devotional from the previous page.*

## MEDITATE:
Reflect upon the content of this devotional. Write, recite and mull over the key verses repeatedly until they reach your heart.

_____
_____
_____
_____

## ENGAGE:
Discuss this devotional with a trusted spiritual friend, pastor or counselor. Share your struggles relating to this devotional. Write whatever significant feedback they offer you. Most importantly, incorporate this devotional into your prayer life.

_____
_____
_____
_____

## DECIDE:
Consider the practical decisions you must make regarding this devotional. Write down those decisions and seek someone to keep you accountable.

_____
_____
_____
_____

## SURVEY:
Take note of your progress regarding this devotional. Changes don't happen suddenly but subtly. Write down any subtle improvements you notice over some time.

_____
_____
_____
_____

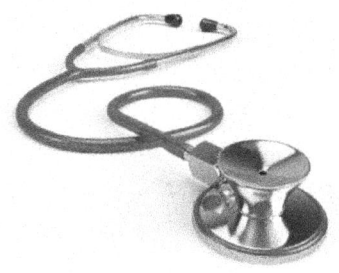

# BIPOLAR:

*Sudden or seasonal changes in a person's moods, energy, and functionality, ranging from mania to depression.*

<u>RELEVANT BIBLICAL PERSONALITIES:</u>
Elijah (I Kings 18:38, I Kings 19)
David (Job 2:1, 11, 20-22, 26)
King Nebuchadnezzar (Daniel 4:33)
Baruch (Jeremiah 45:5)
Fool (Proverbs 17:24)

## MANAGING BIPOLAR DISORDER

*"I discipline my body and keep it under control."*
I Corinthians 9:27

A helium-inflatable without a grounded person holding the string means a balloon floats away into nowhere, eventually crashing when it runs out of air. Likewise, Bipolar illness consists of erratic fluctuations in moods without certain grounding factors such as active faith, a supportive community, a good therapist, and appropriate meds. Amongst these grounding factors, developing temperance sits top of the list. Temperance is the divinely assisted ability (Galatians 5:22) to manage one's impulses at flaring moments. Temperance means saying, "No" to a late-night party that will result in a chocolate binge (or whatever you crave), disrupt your sleep, and arouse your mania. One of the keys to mitigating depressive episodes is tempering your mania. Like the helium-inflatable, you can avoid a reckless crash by staying grounded during an escalating flight.

The largest global M.R.I. study ever conducted on Bipolar illness indicated remarkable differences in people with the disorder. More specifically, the brain regions that regulate impulses were weaker (Hibar et al., 2017). Nonetheless, brain matter is not carved in stone but works like soft clay; it's capable of twisting and turning into new designs. Experts in neuroplasticity, such as Dr. Norman Doidge, taught us that decisions play a substantial role in shaping dispositions through their extensive research. We don't just make choices, but our choices make us.

In our focal passage, the Apostle Paul recognizes the authority God granted him over his own body. The Apostle perceives his flesh as an animal that requires taming or a helium-floatable that warrants grounding. In light of his violent background, I'm sure that the Apostle had to keep many wild impulses in check throughout his day. Yet, we have no record of Post-Damascus Paul ever flying off the handle; instead, he lived a stable, productive life. Paul practiced temperance – stay ground & clutch the string at moments when the fast winds beat against your balloon.

---

**Related Verses:**
*Galatians 5:22, Proverbs 16:32, II Peter 1:6*

# DAILY M.E.D.S.:

*Apply this tool to receive the medicinal benefits of the devotional from the previous page.*

## MEDITATE:
Reflect upon the content of this devotional. Write, recite and mull over the key verses repeatedly until they reach your heart.

_____
_____
_____
_____

## ENGAGE:
Discuss this devotional with a trusted spiritual friend, pastor or counselor. Share your struggles relating to this devotional. Write whatever significant feedback they offer you. Most importantly, incorporate this devotional into your prayer life.

_____
_____
_____
_____

## DECIDE:
Consider the practical decisions you must make regarding this devotional. Write down those decisions and seek someone to keep you accountable.

_____
_____
_____
_____

## SURVEY:
Take note of your progress regarding this devotional. Changes don't happen suddenly but subtly. Write down any subtle improvements you notice over some time.

_____
_____
_____
_____

# THE CHASE FOR HAPPINESS
*"Godliness with contentment is of great gain." I Timothy 6:6*

The pursuit of happiness is like trying to grasp the wet soap bar in the shower. Just when you think you got that sucker in your hands, it's gone! Making happiness an objective hardly ever ends well. Do you want evidence? Take a visit to a furniture store, make comfort your primary focus, and you'll probably find that every chair you sprawl out in strangely becomes uncomfortable. Things like comfort, happiness, and pleasure turn elusive when we hunt for them. The great literary, Nathaniel Hawthorne, paints a picture of this phenomenon perfectly, "Happiness is a butterfly, which when pursued, is always just beyond your grasp. But, if you sit down quietly, it just might land upon you." Perhaps happiness isn't an obtainable objective but an outcome. Folks during manic episodes often chase happiness like running after the elusive butterfly.

Mauss and colleagues (2011) endeavored to answer the question, "Can the pursuit of happiness make people unhappy?". With the bliss and glee of our culture, researchers hypothesized that the goal to be happy backfires on you. Sure enough, they discovered the paradoxical effects amongst a host of female participants. In their study, female participants who placed a high value on happiness showed the least amount of satisfaction when introduced to a happy stimulus. As I said, chairs in a furniture store become uncomfortable the instant you seek comfort. Or, as Hawthorne stated, pursuing happiness is like chasing a butterfly.

The term, contentment, is cold water to the faces of those who pursue happiness. To pursue something means you do NOT have the object of your desire. Yet, the Greek term for contentment in I Timothy 6 is defined as "the perception of your present lot as enough and entire." In other words, contentment means you already have what you need to be fulfilled. The chase (a.k.a. pursuit) is for fools who've come under the illusion of insufficiency. If you want to be happy, heed the Bible's instructions. Take Hawthorne's advice. Sit quietly before the Lord, give thanks for whatever is in your lot, and the butterfly of happiness may find its landing upon your soul. Hard facts, if you don't delight in what you have, you'll never enjoy what you want.

---

**Related Verses:**
*Psalm 37:4 Proverbs 17:24, Matthew 5:1-12*

# DAILY M.E.D.S.:
*Apply this tool to receive the medicinal benefits of the devotional from the previous page.*

## MEDITATE:
Reflect upon the content of this devotional. Write, recite and mull over the key verses repeatedly until they reach your heart.

_____
_____
_____
_____

## ENGAGE:
Discuss this devotional with a trusted spiritual friend, pastor or counselor. Share your struggles relating to this devotional. Write whatever significant feedback they offer you. Most importantly, incorporate this devotional into your prayer life.

_____
_____
_____
_____

## DECIDE:
Consider the practical decisions you must make regarding this devotional. Write down those decisions and seek someone to keep you accountable.

_____
_____
_____
_____

## SURVEY:
Take note of your progress regarding this devotional. Changes don't happen suddenly but subtly. Write down any subtle improvements you notice over some time.

_____
_____
_____
_____

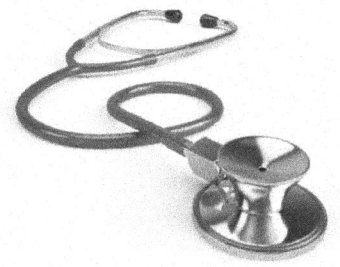

# BORDERLINE PERSONALITY DISORDER:

*A mental health disorder that impacts the way you think and feel about yourself and others, causing problems functioning in everyday life. It includes self-image issues, difficulty managing emotions and behavior, and a pattern of unstable relationships.*

<u>RELEVANT BIBLICAL PERSONALITIES:</u>
Saul (I Samuel 18, 19, 31)
Demoniac Man (Mark:5)
Woman the Well (John 4)

# BORDERLINE PERSONALITY DISORDER & SELF-HATRED

*"The punishment that brought us peace was upon him, and by his wounds we are healed." Isaiah 53:5*

Borderline Personality Disorder (BPD) sufferers are the most likely to commit suicide amongst all mental health disorders. Studies verify that over 70% of BPD sufferers attempt suicide while 10% successfully terminate their existence (that's 400 x the rate of the general population!). Renown Pastor Rick Warren stated that his 27-year-old son, Matthew, battled with BPD for years before his tragic ending. Profound emptiness, chronic fear and an intense self-hatred haunts BPD sufferers like the ghosts that relentlessly stalked Amityville.

Let's square off with a primary factor of BPD - Self-Hatred. A systematic review of all studies relating to BPD from 1980-2006 indicated that 41% of sufferers engaged in at least 50 self-mutilating acts (Oumaya, 2008). These self-mutilating acts include cutting, head banging, reckless driving, substance abuse and a host of other extreme behaviors. Such masochistic tendencies are motivated by the need to solicit the attention of a person they perceive will abandon them and/or an urge to punish oneself for being bad.

Perhaps the greatest promise of the gospel is the scapegoat of Christ. In Old Testament times, the sins of the people were transferred to a scapegoat slaughtered to atone for those sins. On calvary, Jesus became our scapegoat. After Martin Luther (arguably a BPD sufferer) tortured himself for years to atone for his own misdeeds, he came to the realization that his sinfulness necessitated death. Luther allegedly stated, "I must die or someone must die for me." Fortunately, Luther awakened to the fact that Christ already paid the price. His self-mutilation stopped with such a precious revelation. BDP sufferers, take heart - you need not harm yourself since Christ was punished for you

---

## Related Verses:
*Psalm 139:13-14, I Corinthians 6:19-20, Ephesians 1*

# DAILY M.E.D.S.:

*Apply this tool to receive the medicinal benefits of the devotional from the previous page.*

## MEDITATE:
Reflect upon the content of this devotional. Write, recite and mull over the key verses repeatedly until they reach your heart.

_____
_____
_____
_____

## ENGAGE:
Discuss this devotional with a trusted spiritual friend, pastor or counselor. Share your struggles relating to this devotional. Write whatever significant feedback they offer you. Most importantly, incorporate this devotional into your prayer life.

_____
_____
_____
_____

## DECIDE:
Consider the practical decisions you must make regarding this devotional. Write down those decisions and seek someone to keep you accountable.

_____
_____
_____
_____

## SURVEY:
Take note of your progress regarding this devotional. Changes don't happen suddenly but subtly. Write down any subtle improvements you notice over some time.

_____
_____
_____
_____

# BORDERLINE PERSONALITY DISORDER & THE FEAR OF ABANDONMENT

*"I will never leave you nor forsake you."*
*Hebrews 13:5*

Here's an inescapable fact of life – people leave. Like cogs that briefly rub against each other in a cogwheel, we brush up against people who come and go within our lives. People leave to enroll in an out of state college, land better job opportunities, pursue romantic interests and ultimately death. Like the rotation of the cogs, those same folks occasionally return in a later season to touch us one again. But sometimes people don't return; an inevitable part of existence that cannot be eliminated but only tolerated. Not coming to terms with such a harsh reality puts your mental health in jeopardy during moments of abandonment, departure, and death.

The fear of abandonment is widely recognized as a key symptom in diagnosing people with Borderline Personality Disorder. Many sufferers grapple with forming healthy attachments with people since they deeply fear the dissolvement of any close, intimate relationships. In a qualitative study conducted by researchers at the University of Bergen, participants with B.D.P. described the turmoil of belonging to any group. One participant reported intense feelings of anxiety associated with group involvement (Kverme et al., 2019). It's frightening to even say, "hello", when you are haunted by the fact that every "hello" is a prelude to an eventual "goodbye".

The absence of one thing often accentuates our appreciation for the presence of something else. For instance, blind musicians report a greater sensitivity towards sounds, orphans appreciate their teachers and starving people delight in the taste of even a saltine cracker. In the same way, moments of being abandoned by people set the stage for us to relish in the immutable presence of God. Jesus promises all of us, "I will never leave you nor forsake you". This promise is most appreciated when our relationships with people dissolve. In the words of Mother Theresa, "You don't know that God is all you need until God is all you have".

---

### Related Verses:
*Psalm 139:11, Joshua 1:9, Psalm 84:1-2*

# DAILY M.E.D.S.:

*Apply this tool to receive the medicinal benefits of the devotional from the previous page.*

### MEDITATE:
Reflect upon the content of this devotional. Write, recite and mull over the key verses repeatedly until they reach your heart.

_____
_____
_____
_____

### ENGAGE:
Discuss this devotional with a trusted spiritual friend, pastor or counselor. Share your struggles relating to this devotional. Write whatever significant feedback they offer you. Most importantly, incorporate this devotional into your prayer life.

_____
_____
_____
_____

### DECIDE:
Consider the practical decisions you must make regarding this devotional. Write down those decisions and seek someone to keep you accountable.

_____
_____
_____
_____

### SURVEY:
Take note of your progress regarding this devotional. Changes don't happen suddenly but subtly. Write down any subtle improvements you notice over some time.

_____
_____
_____
_____

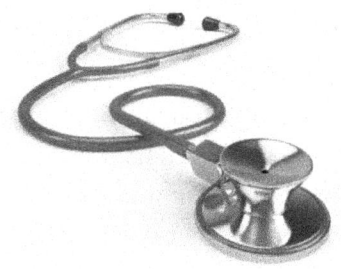

# CODEPENDENCY:

*A loss of one's own personal identity that results in preoccupations with fixing, enabling controlling or being controlled by someone else.*

### RELEVANT BIBLICAL PERSONALITIES:
Rebecca (Genesis 27:5-7)

Mother of James and John (Matthew 20:20-28)

Martha (Luke 10:40)

Eli (I Samuel 2:12-25)

# A FEW POINTERS FOR THOSE WHO STRUGGLE WITH SAYING, "NO"

*Jesus said, "Let your 'Yes' be 'Yes,' and your 'No' be 'No.'" Mt. 5:37*

Chances are, your "No" will be tested by pests, prowlers, and puppeteers who push hard until you cave in on your convictions. Here are a few pointers in saying and staying with your "No."

1. Consider Your Other Commitments

One of the reasons why we struggle with saying "No", is we feel selfish. But in many cases, you're saying "No" so that you don't squander the time and energy required for other commitments. By considering those other commitments - your spouse, your kids, your ministry, etc - you free yourself from the lie that you're selfish. And, you become impervious to guilt trips from folks who try to make you feel selfish as a means of wearing you down enough to say, "Alright, fine!'.

2. Offer Other Options

Given that I hold a PhD in Behavioral Science and pastored for many years, I receive requests all the time from people looking for counseling. I am a teacher, author, minister, consultant, and advocate but NOT a counselor. Instead of saying "No", I typically say, "I'm sorry I can't help you but maybe you should contact my therapist friend." It makes it easier to say "No" to people when I offer them alternatives.

3. Realize your worth

Being unable to establish boundaries is a manifestation of low self-worth. You will never find a high level of security around a junkyard because it doesn't hold much worth. Likewise, people who do not know their worth have very low-security mechanisms (aka boundaries). Conversely, banks have high security because boundaries are enforced where worth is recognized. Know your worth, and saying "No" will be easy.

---

## Related Verses:
*Psalm 16:5-6, Galatians 5:1, Matthew 7:15*

# DAILY M.E.D.S.:

*Apply this tool to receive the medicinal benefits of the devotional from the previous page.*

## MEDITATE:
Reflect upon the content of this devotional. Write, recite and mull over the key verses repeatedly until they reach your heart.

_____
_____
_____
_____

## ENGAGE:
Discuss this devotional with a trusted spiritual friend, pastor or counselor. Share your struggles relating to this devotional. Write whatever significant feedback they offer you. Most importantly, incorporate this devotional into your prayer life.

_____
_____
_____
_____

## DECIDE:
Consider the practical decisions you must make regarding this devotional. Write down those decisions and seek someone to keep you accountable.

_____
_____
_____
_____

## SURVEY:
Take note of your progress regarding this devotional. Changes don't happen suddenly but subtly. Write down any subtle improvements you notice over some time.

_____
_____
_____
_____

# THE FAMILY TRAP

*"Then they scoffed, 'He's just the carpenter's son, and we know Mary, his mother, and his brothers—James, Joseph, Simon, and Judas.'" Matthew 13:55*

Making a break from your family of origin is a critical component of personal growth. Often unintended, snarky siblings, patronizing dads, and smothering moms are millstones that weigh us down. For this reason, it is not uncommon within the scriptures for God to command His Chosen Ones to leave their kinfolk for at least a little while. He instructs Abraham to take a break from his father's household (Genesis 12:1), Jeremiah to bolt from his hometown Anathoth (Jeremiah 1), and Jesus to back up from Joseph and Mary (Luke 2:49). Attention, you who are cradled and coddled, coming into your own always begins by coming out of your home.

According to Family Systems Theory, a model of social psychology, family unit members intimately network together like parts of a body. Just as the hand cannot operate without the arm, a person cannot function without the support of their relatives. Now, for a SEASON, this is necessary for our early development, just like the caterpillar requires its cocoon and the baby eagle its nest. But, beyond that season, the place that trained you morphs into a place that traps you. Your family can become a trap.

So, Jesus visits the old neighborhood. We see that the most outstanding man ever born was nothing more than "a carpenter's son" within that familiar region. Sad to say, but the last people on earth to recognize that you're exceptional will be the people from whom you are the exception. If Jesus never left his old stomping grounds, he may have been affected by their small opinion of him. If Jesus never made a break from being the Son of Mary, He may have never come into the fullness of being the Son of God. Once again, coming into your own means first coming out of your home.

---

### Related Verses:
*Genesis 12:1, Luke 2:49, Matthew 10:14*

Dr. JESUS

# DAILY M.E.D.S.:
*Apply this tool to receive the medicinal benefits of the devotional from the previous page.*

## MEDITATE:
Reflect upon the content of this devotional. Write, recite and mull over the key verses repeatedly until they reach your heart.

_____
_____
_____
_____

## ENGAGE:
Discuss this devotional with a trusted spiritual friend, pastor or counselor. Share your struggles relating to this devotional. Write whatever significant feedback they offer you. Most importantly, incorporate this devotional into your prayer life.

_____
_____
_____
_____

## DECIDE:
Consider the practical decisions you must make regarding this devotional. Write down those decisions and seek someone to keep you accountable.

_____
_____
_____
_____

## SURVEY:
Take note of your progress regarding this devotional. Changes don't happen suddenly but subtly. Write down any subtle improvements you notice over some time.

_____
_____
_____
_____

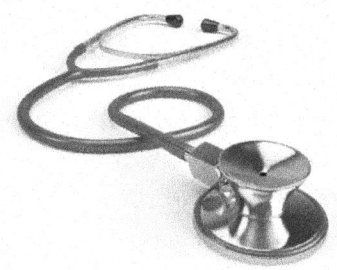

# CRISIS:

*An experience with an event is an intolerable difficulty that exceeds the person's current resources and coping mechanisms.*

<u>RELEVANT BIBLICAL PERSONALITIES:</u>
Job (Job 1:13-22)
Solomon (Ecclesiastes 1:14)
Jesus (Matthew 26:36-46)
Noah (Genesis 6:9-9:17)
Good Samaritan & Half-Dead Man (Luke 10:25-37)

# A CRISIS & THE GOSPEL

*"When he came to his senses, he said, 'How many of my father's hired servants have food to spare, and here I am starving to death!'" Luke 15:17*

The gospel only became edible when I was sleeping on a loose mattress within the hallway of an overpopulated juvenile detention center, crammed up against bandits, slayers, and gangbangers. That's my story! If I heard the sermon a few months prior while joyriding in a stolen car, laughing up life w/ homies, I would've undoubtedly choked on its demands. Pastor Mike, the tender-hearted, tough-guy minister and staff member of the juvenile detention center, shared Jesus with me at an opportunistic moment of utter loneliness. His seed germinated deeply, only because a storm ravished my calloused heart. A good thing about natural disasters is that they soften the hard ground. In happy times, a man smugly spits out the truths of Christ with an attitude; in hairy times, he swallows them with gratitude. A crisis is what makes the gospel digestible to an otherwise resistant soul.

Three types of crisis happen during the journey called life. First, a developmental crisis is defined as the struggles that accompany any kind of growth from puberty to promotions, a.k.a., "growing pains" (read Erikson's stages of development). Second, an existential crisis is defined as the conflicts that happen quietly within the soul regarding the meaning of life (read Ecclesiastes). Third, a situational crisis is when trouble suddenly befalls you through an accident or a catastrophe (read the newspaper). The one common denominator between all three crises is what Sir Isaac Newton articulated in the second law of motion, "everything remains in a state of inertia until thrust upon by some outward force". Crisis, no matter what kind, is a motivator for change.

A second glance at the Prodigal Son's classic statement enlightens us to the fact that a crisis prompts his repentance. Without a famine, he might never come to his senses. Moms and dads - if circumstances worsened since you started pleading with heaven for your child, rejoice in answered prayer. Contrary to popular opinion, the prodigal son didn't return home because he was sorry; he went home because he was hungry. His famine crisis is what wooed him back to the Father's house. A crisis is a prelude to homecoming.

---

## Related Verses:
*Isaiah 45:7, Romans 5:3-5, John 16:33*

# DAILY M.E.D.S.:
*Apply this tool to receive the medicinal benefits of the devotional from the previous page.*

### MEDITATE:
Reflect upon the content of this devotional. Write, recite and mull over the key verses repeatedly until they reach your heart.

_____
_____
_____
_____

### ENGAGE:
Discuss this devotional with a trusted spiritual friend, pastor or counselor. Share your struggles relating to this devotional. Write whatever significant feedback they offer you. Most importantly, incorporate this devotional into your prayer life.

_____
_____
_____
_____

### DECIDE:
Consider the practical decisions you must make regarding this devotional. Write down those decisions and seek someone to keep you accountable.

_____
_____
_____
_____

### SURVEY:
Take note of your progress regarding this devotional. Changes don't happen suddenly but subtly. Write down any subtle improvements you notice over some time.

_____
_____
_____
_____

# VICARIOUS CRISIS

*"Let each of you look not only to his own interests,
but also to the interests of others." Philippians 2:4.*

What would you do if you heard a young woman screaming bloody murder on a city street? "I'd rush to her aid, assail her attackers, or at least call 911", I suppose. Of course, I'd like to believe that I'm Liam Neeson. But, in Philippians 2:4, the Apostle recognizes that we must hurdle over a host of self-interests when deciding to help someone in a jam. The answer to the question is not as simple as you suppose. Latane and Darley (1968) were two behavioral scientists who proposed a theory that lays out all the mental hurdles we must overcome before deciding to help someone in an emergency. Your response to these five critical questions determines whether or not you would respond rightly to an emergency.

### 1. DO YOU NOTICE THE EMERGENCY?
Considering the cell phone in your hands, the worries on your mind, and all of the sounds of city traffic, you might not even notice such an ordeal.

### 2. DO YOU SEE IT AS AN EMERGENCY?
Because few bystanders in the vicinity appear distressed, a possibility surfaces that you might dismiss the incident as a hoax by taking cues from the crowds.

### 3. DO YOU ASSUME RESPONSIBILITY?
Considering the reality that there are so many other people nearby, a possibility emerges that you might diffuse responsibility – "someone else will take care of it."

### 4. DO YOU KNOW THE RIGHT RESPONSE?
You might stall out of mental confusion since your mind rushes in a thousand directions when under pressure.

### 5. DO YOU HAVE THE COURAGE TO ACT?
Because 2 out of 4 survival instincts are usually counterproductive in these circumstances (flight and freeze), a possibility arises that you'd be too afraid to act.

---

## Related Verses:
*Luke 10:25-37, James 4:17, Psalm 41:1*

# DAILY M.E.D.S.:

*Apply this tool to receive the medicinal benefits of the devotional from the previous page.*

### MEDITATE:
Reflect upon the content of this devotional. Write, recite and mull over the key verses repeatedly until they reach your heart.

_____
_____
_____
_____

### ENGAGE:
Discuss this devotional with a trusted spiritual friend, pastor or counselor. Share your struggles relating to this devotional. Write whatever significant feedback they offer you. Most importantly, incorporate this devotional into your prayer life.

_____
_____
_____
_____

### DECIDE:
Consider the practical decisions you must make regarding this devotional. Write down those decisions and seek someone to keep you accountable.

_____
_____
_____
_____

### SURVEY:
Take note of your progress regarding this devotional. Changes don't happen suddenly but subtly. Write down any subtle improvements you notice over some time.

_____
_____
_____
_____

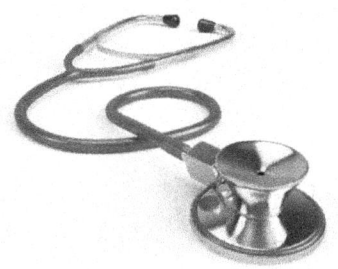

# DEPRESSION:

*Characterized by persistent sadness and a loss of interest in formerly pleasurable activities along with significant impairment in life.*

RELEVANT BIBLICAL PERSONALITIES:
Elijah (I Kings 19)
David (Psalm 6)
Heman Son of Korah (Psalm 88)
Jeremiah (Lamentations 2:10)

## AN EYE FOR WHAT'S GOOD

*"Open their eyes and turn them from darkness to light
and from the power of Satan to God..." Acts 26:18*

Sadly, bad is more potent than good, at least in our heads. For instance, a social experiment was performed that indicated that participants' distress who lost $50 was more significant than the pleasure of participants who gained $50. Sheldon, Ryan, and Reis (1996) conducted studies that reveal you're more likely to remember a bad than a good yesterday. The proverbial powers of darkness hijack way too much of our attention, especially amongst those who suffer from depression.

We often miss a good thing when it shows up in our midst. In 2007, over 1,090 D.C. residents snubbed a disheveled man playing the violin inside the Metro train station. Only a handful of people stopped for a brief time to listen to the man's song. Unbeknownst to Washington D.C., the man was legendary violinist, Joshua Bell, playing one of the most sophisticated tunes on a violin worth 3.5 million dollars. The violinist was recruited by sociologists experimenting on humanity's perception of beauty, and we failed miserably. Now, if Charles Manson were reading Tarot cards in that same Metro Train station, a crowd would have gathered larger than Yankee Stadium.

Perhaps one of the most fantastic promises in the bible is God opening our spiritual eyes, as stated in Acts 26:18. Our fallen condition (the state of affairs resultant from sin) is such that not only do we fail to spot the awesome, but we are preoccupied with the awful. Nothing short of an absolute miracle transpires, as recorded in Acts 26:18 when we transition from noticing diabolical activities to divine happenings. In your marriage, within the lives of your children, amongst your superiors and subordinates, shall you see God today. May we all be able to say, "I was once blind, but now I see."

### Related Verses:
*Romans 12:9, Matthew 5:8, John 9:25*

# DAILY M.E.D.S.:

*Apply this tool to receive the medicinal benefits of the devotional from the previous page.*

## MEDITATE:
Reflect upon the content of this devotional. Write, recite and mull over the key verses repeatedly until they reach your heart.

_____
_____
_____
_____

## ENGAGE:
Discuss this devotional with a trusted spiritual friend, pastor or counselor. Share your struggles relating to this devotional. Write whatever significant feedback they offer you. Most importantly, incorporate this devotional into your prayer life.

_____
_____
_____
_____

## DECIDE:
Consider the practical decisions you must make regarding this devotional. Write down those decisions and seek someone to keep you accountable.

_____
_____
_____
_____

## SURVEY:
Take note of your progress regarding this devotional. Changes don't happen suddenly but subtly. Write down any subtle improvements you notice over some time.

_____
_____
_____
_____

DEPRESSION

# THE PSYCHOLOGY OF PRAISE
*"The LORD answered, 'Judah shall go up first; I have given the land into their hands.'" Judges 1:2.*

Chances are the first part of your body to react to any sudden disaster is your mouth. Stub your toe, and watch your tongue run loose like a wild horse. A nearby car almost sideswipes you, and you watch your mouth drop bombs like August 6, 1945. Foolishly, we presume that we can superintend an ordeal by verbally condemning it. Instead, we find that our cursing and complaining don't eliminate but only escalates our problems. Parents who criticize their rebellious children discover their behaviors only amplifying. Employees who vent about their workplace drama become more frustrated. Conversely, a mouth that sounds off praise amidst the battle preps the mind for victory.

In Judges 1, Yahweh commands His people to "send Judah first" - the division of the army that consisted of singing soldiers. Through this instruction, Yahweh teaches His people about the power of praise amidst the battles of life. Research shows that praising God may not change what you're going through, but it most definitely alters what's going through you. In a study conducted on 1,024 adults across the United States, singing religious music was shown to release certain neurotransmitters that enhance our sense of control over disarray (Bradshaw et al., 2015). Feelings of helplessness and hopelessness go down as the praises go up. This finding is significant for people with depression since depression often consists of helplessness. Let me break it down for you like this....

Two baby frogs mistakenly plunge into a bowl of cream. The first frog sounds off his complaints, "How the heck we getting out of here! Now, we're doomed!". Betwixt his words, he guzzled a fatal dose of cream, drowning to death. The second frog resolved not to say one single statement about his predicament. Instead, he started swimming while quietly singing. "I'll make the best of this life", he thought while moving and grooving. After a few minutes, the cream churned into a hard stick of butter from all the frog's motions. There, the frog stood on top of the butter with a champion's smile. When you can't see your way out, sing your way out.

---

## Related Verses:
*Philippians 4:4-8, Psalm 150:1-6, Psalm 42:5*

# DAILY M.E.D.S.:

*Apply this tool to receive the medicinal benefits of the devotional from the previous page.*

## MEDITATE:
Reflect upon the content of this devotional. Write, recite and mull over the key verses repeatedly until they reach your heart.

_____
_____
_____
_____

## ENGAGE:
Discuss this devotional with a trusted spiritual friend, pastor or counselor. Share your struggles relating to this devotional. Write whatever significant feedback they offer you. Most importantly, incorporate this devotional into your prayer life.

_____
_____
_____
_____

## DECIDE:
Consider the practical decisions you must make regarding this devotional. Write down those decisions and seek someone to keep you accountable.

_____
_____
_____
_____

## SURVEY:
Take note of your progress regarding this devotional. Changes don't happen suddenly but subtly. Write down any subtle improvements you notice over some time.

_____
_____
_____
_____

# EMBRACE THE SURPRISES:
# A KEY TO DEFEATING DEPRESSION

*"For your daughter-in-law, Ruth is better to you than seven sons, and she has given birth. Then Naomi took Ruth's child in her arms and cared for him." Ruth 4:16*

The depressed psyche is cemented with "should" fixations. For instance, "I should be married by now," "I should have finished college," "My mom should be here," "I should have known what was happening to my child," and the violin plays on. These "should" fixations are hatched by idealism, a grandiose philosophy that says, "Life must be a certain way, and I won't accept it any other way." Clark Griswold from Christmas Vacation is the classic idealist losing his mental faculties from pursuing "should(s)" that shall never happen. "The Christmas lights should work!", "Everyone should be together for the holidays!", "I should get a huge Christmas bonus this year!", etc. All kidding aside, this should-mentality is a breeding ground for mental illness. The idealistic mind breaks down quickly since it has no flexibility, just like glass shatters because it has no elasticity.

Uncovering depression, you'll find inflexible idealism at its core. In more than 20 years of research, Gordon Flett, Ph.D. indicated strong correlations between perfectionism and depression. According to Flett, folks with depression have trouble coping with circumstances that don't match the utopia within their minds. Sometimes, depression manifests with shaking your fists, "I hate life!". Other times, depression manifests with throwing your hands up, "I give up! I just can't win!". Either way, whether mad or sad, depression prevails whenever you demand what life should be. Conversely, embracing what "shall be" rather than demanding what "should be" paves a way out of a pit.

Regarding our passage of study, giving birth to "sons" is a dream come true for every Hebrew mother. Naomi is severely depressed (so depressed she changed her name to Mara which means "bitter") because that dream was crushed when her sons were killed by catastrophe. Naomi lives most of her life grieving shattered ideals rather than embracing new realities. Suddenly, her eyes open to the fact that although life didn't pan out the way it was planned out, it trumped her ideals. God says, "Ruth (and Ruth's baby) is better to you than seven sons," which translates to, "What shall happen will be even better than what you thought should happen." Depression lessens when you learn this lesson - Life's greatest gifts are not what you planned or imagined but often take you by surprise. Open yourself up to the surprises, Clark!

---

## Related Verses:
*Ephesians 3:20, Psalm 37:4, Jeremiah 29:11*

# DAILY M.E.D.S.:

*Apply this tool to receive the medicinal benefits of the devotional from the previous page.*

## MEDITATE:
Reflect upon the content of this devotional. Write, recite and mull over the key verses repeatedly until they reach your heart.

_____
_____
_____
_____

## ENGAGE:
Discuss this devotional with a trusted spiritual friend, pastor or counselor. Share your struggles relating to this devotional. Write whatever significant feedback they offer you. Most importantly, incorporate this devotional into your prayer life.

_____
_____
_____
_____

## DECIDE:
Consider the practical decisions you must make regarding this devotional. Write down those decisions and seek someone to keep you accountable.

_____
_____
_____
_____

## SURVEY:
Take note of your progress regarding this devotional. Changes don't happen suddenly but subtly. Write down any subtle improvements you notice over some time.

_____
_____
_____
_____

# UPBEAT RELATIONSHIPS:
# A KEY TO DEFEATING DEPRESSION
*"Kind words are good medicine...." Proverbs 15:4.*

Moods are contagions you catch from the company you keep. There are two kinds of people in your life – UPPERS and DOWNERS. UPPERS are typically glad until something makes them sad, whereas DOWNERS are usually sad in need of something to make them glad. The first group spreads cheer WHERE-EVER they go, whereas the second group spreads cheer WHENEVER they go. Please don't fool yourself; your emotional make-up is not as watertight as you presume. Instead, your psyche is highly absorbent, affected by the energy others emit. Chill with UPPERS long enough, and you'll feel like you had a shot of B-Vitamin; hence, the proverb, "Kind words are like medicine."

Conversely, hang out with DOWNERS long enough, and you'll secretly wish you got hit with a sledgehammer. Depression is a vibe that partly stems from mingling with a gloomy tribe. A recent study on adolescent depression uncovered the familial characteristics that trigger mental illness symptoms amongst teens. Interestingly enough, it was found that "low affect" from loved ones was a trigger for depression (Pereira et al., 2015). Examples of low affect include a lack of enthusiasm when sharing your dreams, a deficiency of warmth when you're hurting, and a negatively aloof attitude towards your overall existence. Few things crush you like a blank stare and eyes glazed with disinterest from family and friends at a moment when your heart is cracked wide open.

Defeating depression doesn't mean defriending all the DOWNERS in your life - God no! You were strategically situated in dark places to shine brightly. DOWNERS are often the missions field God calls you to reach with the love of Christ. Where would they be without your presence? Instead, defeating depression means investing enough time with UPPERS to offset the expense of being with DOWNERS. Mathematically speaking, your account bounces if there are more withdrawals than deposits. UPPERS make deposits that keep your books (a.k.a., your head) balanced. Never underestimate the rejuvenation that occurs over a cup of coffee with an upbeat friend. Cherish the UPPERS in your life, those listed on the acknowledgment page of your survivor's manual.

---

## Related Verses:
*Ecclesiastes 4:9-12, Proverbs 13:20, II Corinthians 6:14*

Dr. JESUS

# DAILY M.E.D.S.:
*Apply this tool to receive the medicinal benefits of the devotional from the previous page.*

## MEDITATE:
Reflect upon the content of this devotional. Write, recite and mull over the key verses repeatedly until they reach your heart.

_____
_____
_____
_____

## ENGAGE:
Discuss this devotional with a trusted spiritual friend, pastor or counselor. Share your struggles relating to this devotional. Write whatever significant feedback they offer you. Most importantly, incorporate this devotional into your prayer life.

_____
_____
_____
_____

## DECIDE:
Consider the practical decisions you must make regarding this devotional. Write down those decisions and seek someone to keep you accountable.

_____
_____
_____
_____

## SURVEY:
Take note of your progress regarding this devotional. Changes don't happen suddenly but subtly. Write down any subtle improvements you notice over some time.

_____
_____
_____
_____

## HUMILITY: A KEY IN DEFEATING DEPRESSION
*"Humble yourself before the Lord, and He will lift you up." James 4:10*

Depression frequently works in tandem with self-absorption. A narrow spotlight zeroes in on MY feelings, MY past, MY mistakes, MY losses, MY hurts, while blacking out the picturesque scenery on all sides. Many years ago, a depressed fella divulged to me during a pastoral counseling session, "It's Christmas morning, my beautiful wife smiles, my kids laugh, we live comfortably, and yet I can't get out of my own dark head." Studies show that folks with depression overuse personal pronouns such as "I", "Me" and "My" within their speech while hardly ever uttering, "We", "He" or "She" (Petsko, 2018). Textual analysis conducted on Kurt Cobain and Sylvia Plath (both poets who committed suicide) reveal an over-saturation of personal pronouns. Ample studies confirm the unholy, synergetic alliance between depression and self-absorption.

Some say, "Depression paves the way for self-absorption". Pain is like a bratty child that demands our full attention. You could be sprawled out on a Bahamas beach while chit-chatting with your favorite company. But if you have a throbbing toothache, it's a tricky thing to focus on anything other than your fangs. Pain, whether physical or emotional, holds our focus hostage! Others say, "Self-absorption paves the way for depression." Alleviating a particular agony by simply putting your mind on something outside of yourself is a common experience for most of us. Facts are, determining what paves the way for the other is as silly as trying to figure out if the right or left foot leads your body while walking.

The Apostle James offers a promise for anyone in a pit. How you landed in the pit (whether it's because you are self-addicted or just afflicted) is not as significant as how you will be lifted out of the pit. According to the text, "humble yourself before the Lord, and He will lift you up." Humbling yourself does NOT mean thinking less of yourself (Eg. "I'm such a worm!"), but rather thinking of yourself less. Humbling yourself before the Lord equates to getting so vacuumed into the grandness of God that you forget the smallness of your existence. Few things refute being overwhelmed by your pain like being overtaken by your God.

---

### Related Verses:
*I Corinthians 10:26, Proverbs 11:25, II Chronicles 7:14*

# DAILY M.E.D.S.:

*Apply this tool to receive the medicinal benefits of the devotional from the previous page.*

## MEDITATE:
Reflect upon the content of this devotional. Write, recite and mull over the key verses repeatedly until they reach your heart.

_____
_____
_____
_____

## ENGAGE:
Discuss this devotional with a trusted spiritual friend, pastor or counselor. Share your struggles relating to this devotional. Write whatever significant feedback they offer you. Most importantly, incorporate this devotional into your prayer life.

_____
_____
_____
_____

## DECIDE:
Consider the practical decisions you must make regarding this devotional. Write down those decisions and seek someone to keep you accountable.

_____
_____
_____
_____

## SURVEY:
Take note of your progress regarding this devotional. Changes don't happen suddenly but subtly. Write down any subtle improvements you notice over some time.

_____
_____
_____
_____

# GET IT OFF YOUR CHEST: A KEY TO DEFEATING DEPRESSION

*"When I kept silent, my bones wasted away through my groaning all day long. For day and night, your hand (God) was heavy on me; my strength was sapped as in the heat of summer. But, then I acknowledged my sin to you..." Psalm 32:3*

Guilt acts like a hefty weight that crushes the soul into shards. Heavy is the adjective applied in describing the conscience plagued by yesterday's crimes - we often say, "a heavy conscience." To prove this is more than a metaphor, Princeton University researchers conducted a study on guilt's impact upon subjective body weight. Researchers discovered that participants who were asked to simply recall a recent sin (such as lying, cheating, or stealing) guesstimated that their physical body weight was heavier than their actual weight. Researchers compared these findings with a control group that didn't recall any sins and calculated their weight lesser (Day, Bobocel, 2012). When the Psalmist pens, "my strength was sapped as in the heat of summer", he describes a common experience amongst those who carry guilt.

Depressed people are often pent-up with secrets - secret struggles, secret feelings, secret sins. Secrecy keeps guilt alive and well, and guilt drags you down. Many therapists report depressed patients recovering from their sadness by merely affording them space to get their sins "off their chest." Harboring unconfessed sins is a sure recipe for emotional depletion that feels much like "depression." As they say in the halls of Alcoholics Anonymous, "you're only as sick as your secrets."

Some suppose, "Don't bother confessing your sins unless you're willing to turn from them." Albeit confession is incomplete without repentance, taking the first step of any task makes it simpler to follow through with subsequent steps. It is easier for a person to arise from a fall after a weight is removed from their chest than trying to regain ground with that burden still on them. In other words, a man is more capable of repentance when the albatross of guilt does not weigh him down. In summary, confession (to Christ and the Body of Christ) paves the way out of a morally induced depression.

---

### Related Verses:
*James 5:16, Proverbs 28:13, I John 1:19*

# DAILY M.E.D.S.:

*Apply this tool to receive the medicinal benefits of the devotional from the previous page.*

### MEDITATE:
Reflect upon the content of this devotional. Write, recite and mull over the key verses repeatedly until they reach your heart.

_____
_____
_____
_____

### ENGAGE:
Discuss this devotional with a trusted spiritual friend, pastor or counselor. Share your struggles relating to this devotional. Write whatever significant feedback they offer you. Most importantly, incorporate this devotional into your prayer life.

_____
_____
_____
_____

### DECIDE:
Consider the practical decisions you must make regarding this devotional. Write down those decisions and seek someone to keep you accountable.

_____
_____
_____
_____

### SURVEY:
Take note of your progress regarding this devotional. Changes don't happen suddenly but subtly. Write down any subtle improvements you notice over some time.

_____
_____
_____
_____

# GO BACK HOME: A KEY IN DEFEATING DEPRESSION

*"Then the Lord God took the man and placed him in the Garden to watch after it." Genesis 2:15.*

Melancholy is the likely response of any species plucked out of its natural habitat. Zoologists report that monkeys in cages are downcast compared to primates in the Jungle (evident by less zest in their steps and heads hunkered down). Like the baboon, we homo-sapiens were plucked out of our natural habitat. God whittled our souls for "the garden,"; an alfresco locale with lots of sunshine, floral scents, and gorgeous greenery. Instead, we inhabit sheet-rocked shanties painted with chemical colors and eyes tranced by virtual realities. We are outside our habitat, spending all our time in office buildings, automobiles, and in front of screens. Make no mistake about it, "we're not in Kansas anymore."

A frequent pilgrimage to our natural habitat is a key in mending our melancholy. Of course, it's an oversimplification to presume nature-walks alone is the cure for the multi-headed Monster known as depression. However, Harvard researchers indicated that 90-minute nature walks (per day) dramatically lowered negative ruminations seen on prefrontal cortex scans (Strauss, 2015). According to Dr. Strauss, the depressed brain is stuck making harmful neurological loops, and nature interrupts that loop. Also, stats indicate that urban-dwellers are 40% more likely to have a mood disorder than rural inhabitants (Weaver, 2013). Even the Psalmist said, "I would have despaired if I had not seen the goodness of God in the LAND of the living"; the Hebrew term land refers, not to a cemented parking lot, but God's green earth.

What keeps us stuck in our sophisticated shanties? Like the monkeys of the zoo, we become acclimated to our surroundings. Acclimation means making psychological adjustments to cope with a new set of circumstances. Just like the primates, we've accepted our new surroundings as normal, but we've lost the zest in our steps. Let us not forget – God made us from the dirt and placed us in a garden. It is only logical, and biblical, that a return to our home of earth boosts our dopamine levels. It doesn't matter if you're surrounded by snow-capped mountains, trees with foliage, or a front lawn that looks like Fenway; consistent exposure to nature of any kind stabilizes your psyches. Feel better by going back home. Take a nature walk at least once a day for 90 minutes.

---

### Related Verses:
*Romans 1:20, Matthew 6:26-28, Proverbs 8:29*

# DAILY M.E.D.S.:
*Apply this tool to receive the medicinal benefits of the devotional from the previous page.*

## MEDITATE:
Reflect upon the content of this devotional. Write, recite and mull over the key verses repeatedly until they reach your heart.

___
___
___
___

## ENGAGE:
Discuss this devotional with a trusted spiritual friend, pastor or counselor. Share your struggles relating to this devotional. Write whatever significant feedback they offer you. Most importantly, incorporate this devotional into your prayer life.

___
___
___
___

## DECIDE:
Consider the practical decisions you must make regarding this devotional. Write down those decisions and seek someone to keep you accountable.

___
___
___
___

## SURVEY:
Take note of your progress regarding this devotional. Changes don't happen suddenly but subtly. Write down any subtle improvements you notice over some time.

___
___
___
___

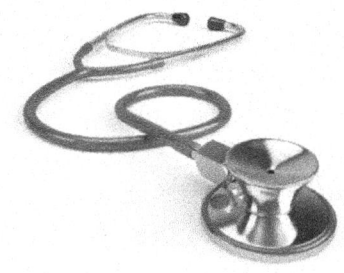

# EATING DISORDER:

*Any range of physiological disorders characterized by abnormal or disturbed eating habits.*

RELEVANT BIBLICAL PERSONALITIES:
King Nebuchadnezzar (Daniel 1:3-16)
Corinthians (I Corinthians 11:33)
Saul (I Samuel 14:24-46)
Elijah (I Kings 19:8)

# BODY IMAGE, SOCIAL COMPARISONS & EATING DISORDERS

*"But when they measure themselves by one another and compare themselves with one another, they are unwise." II Corinthians 10:12*

Applying the wrong-sized tool when fastening a screw leads to 'stripping'. I've stripped many screws using the wrong screwdriver. Each tool is uniquely crafted for a particular task, and utilizing that tool incorrectly only damages whatever you are fixing. Like the tools, you were distinctively composed by God to execute a specific purpose, fit in with particular tribes, marry a specific mate, prefer certain music and express particular views. You were not designed to work anywhere and everywhere. Trying to make yourself like someone else through social comparisons (eg., "I wish I was a good singer like her") is as ludicrous as employing the wrong size tool for a job. Such behavior leads to the 'stripping' of your dignity and self-worth. We do more damage to ourselves than any person could ever inflict upon us with their nasty insults.

Behavioral scientists conducted a study amongst 232 college women that indicated a correlation between social comparisons and eating disorders (Fitzsimmons-Craft, 2017). Two types of social comparisons were examined – upward and downward comparisons. An upward comparison makes you feel inferior by measuring yourself against people you deem as better, whereas a downward comparison makes you feel superior by measuring yourself against people you regard as lesser. Upward comparisons were shown to impact eating pathology. The more women compared themselves with ladies they considered superior, the more they engaged in disorderly eating.

Within our focal passage, the Apostle Paul describes social comparisons as "unwise." The adjective "unwise" applies to any practice that results in the detriment of oneself. For instance, it's unwise to poke a sleeping bear, scoop fire in your lap or use a chainsaw to cut glass. Anticipate all these practices resulting in injury or possible death. With one word, the Apostle warns about the masochistic nature of comparing yourself to your peers. Social comparisons strip you of personal value. Disorderly eating is the patch-up job to masquerade the damage you did to yourself.

---

**Related Verses:**
*John 21:22, Romans 14:17, Romans 12:1*

Dr. JESUS

# DAILY M.E.D.S.:
*Apply this tool to receive the medicinal benefits of the devotional from the previous page.*

## MEDITATE:
Reflect upon the content of this devotional. Write, recite and mull over the key verses repeatedly until they reach your heart.

___
___
___
___

## ENGAGE:
Discuss this devotional with a trusted spiritual friend, pastor or counselor. Share your struggles relating to this devotional. Write whatever significant feedback they offer you. Most importantly, incorporate this devotional into your prayer life.

___
___
___
___

## DECIDE:
Consider the practical decisions you must make regarding this devotional. Write down those decisions and seek someone to keep you accountable.

___
___
___
___

## SURVEY:
Take note of your progress regarding this devotional. Changes don't happen suddenly but subtly. Write down any subtle improvements you notice over some time.

___
___
___
___

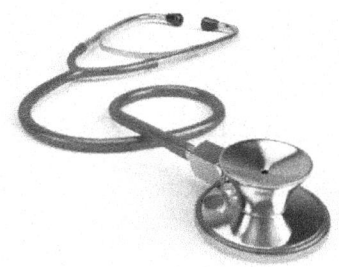

# FATIGUE:

*A state of continual tiredness and/or burnout with diminishing functionality.*

## RELEVANT BIBLICAL PERSONALITIES:
David's Men (I Samuel 30:10, 21-24)

Esau (Genesis 25:29)

Epaphroditus (Philippians 2:25-30)

Disciples (Luke 22:45)

## WATCH OUT FOR WEARINESS
*"He gives strength to the weary..." Isaiah 49:21*

Heavyweight champion George Foreman's lead-loaded punch, validated by an 89% knockout rate, made him a stronger contender than Muhammad Ali on 11/30/74 at the Rumble in the Jungle. All of the boxing pundits knew that night Foreman was stronger. But Ali was smarter. The "psyche you out" Ali used his infamous Rope-A-Dope tactic to make Foreman weary by welcoming endless punches while resting against the ropes. Perfectly timed, Ali retaliated with a strike that banked on Foreman's exhaustion for a sure knockout. Simply stated, Ali won the match by making the champion "weary." Like Foreman, we believers have an opportunistic enemy who waits for us to grow weary before unloading his knockout punch. Watch out for weariness!

In an intriguing study on fatigue and folly, behavioral scientists analyzed 1,100 decisions of magistrates in an Arab court over one year. The researchers concluded that the magistrates made the worse judgments after 4:25pm, a point where the magistrates were exhausted from hearing cases all day (Levav, Stanford University, 2011). Other neuroscientific studies show that fatigue compromises the Temporoparietal Junction, a region of your brain required for sound social judgments. Samson's foolishness with Delilah, David's idiocy with Bathsheba, and Esau's stupidity with Jacob happen at an instant of exhaustion. Make no mistake about it, the smartest people make the stupidest decisions when weary.

Like Foreman, we're up against an opponent rope-a-doping us into throwing futile punches. Nursing resentments, senseless arguing, vindictive backbiting, chronic worry, and chasing fantasies are just a few examples of being rope-a-doped into weariness. All these sinful practices deplete you of your spiritual vitality. Be not deceived because your adversary waits for the zenith of your exhaustion to unload his knockout punch. Perhaps it's time to head back to your coach in the corner for some wisdom on how to fight smarter before your weariness ends in a knockout.

### Related Verses:
*Matthew 11:28-30, Psalm 23:2, Isaiah 40:31*

Dr. JESUS

# DAILY M.E.D.S.:
*Apply this tool to receive the medicinal benefits of the devotional from the previous page.*

### MEDITATE:
Reflect upon the content of this devotional. Write, recite and mull over the key verses repeatedly until they reach your heart.

_____
_____
_____

### ENGAGE:
Discuss this devotional with a trusted spiritual friend, pastor or counselor. Share your struggles relating to this devotional. Write whatever significant feedback they offer you. Most importantly, incorporate this devotional into your prayer life.

_____
_____
_____

### DECIDE:
Consider the practical decisions you must make regarding this devotional. Write down those decisions and seek someone to keep you accountable.

_____
_____
_____

### SURVEY:
Take note of your progress regarding this devotional. Changes don't happen suddenly but subtly. Write down any subtle improvements you notice over some time.

_____
_____
_____

# LIGHTEN YOUR LOADS

*"Come to me all you who are heavy-burdened, and I will give you rest.*
*Take my yoke upon you and learn from me. For my yoke is easy and burden is light."*
Matthew 11:28-30

Animals become tired on the farm, not just from the work they execute but from the load they carry. If an animal lugs heavy burdens, the beast grows tired from something as simple as eating grass. Likewise, we burn out not just from the work we do but also from the mental loads we carry. If you're cashing out customers at a register, you probably won't get too tired after a few hours. But if you're cashing out customers while worrying about your spouse's alcohol problem, or your daughter's failing marriage, or whatever else, just a few minutes of work drain you faster than the holidays deplete your savings account. So, before you quit your job, or step down from that ministry position, under the assumption it's causing fatigue, think again. It might not be the work that's draining you, but the load you're shouldering while working.

Carrying heavy mental loads causes your Amygdala to work overtime. The Amygdala is the part of your brain that reacts to a crisis with appropriate fight-flight responses. The Amygdala is a gift from God that enables you to handle a crisis swiftly and sagaciously. But, keeping the Amygdala active all the time is like firing your weapon whenever you're frightened by a shadow; eventually, you run out of ammunition. In the same way, those who operate their Amygdala every moment of the day, in constant crisis mode, run out of energy.

In our focal passage, Jesus encourages us to assume His burden as a means of overcoming fatigue. He describes His burden as being "light". The term, burden, signifies the mindset of the Savior who stayed fast asleep in a boat during the middle of a sea storm. He's saying, "Let my mind be in you! A mentality that remains lighthearted even during the most difficult days." Whenever I travel on airplanes, I always pack light. I've learned that heavy luggage hinders me from making headway and makes every journey exhausting. Fatigue is often the indication that it's time to unload your burdens at the feet of Jesus so that you can travel light.

---

**Related Verses:**
*I Peter 5:7, Mark 4:38-40, Psalm 94:19*

Dr. JESUS

# DAILY M.E.D.S.:
*Apply this tool to receive the medicinal benefits of the devotional from the previous page.*

### MEDITATE:
Reflect upon the content of this devotional. Write, recite and mull over the key verses repeatedly until they reach your heart.

___
___
___
___

### ENGAGE:
Discuss this devotional with a trusted spiritual friend, pastor or counselor. Share your struggles relating to this devotional. Write whatever significant feedback they offer you. Most importantly, incorporate this devotional into your prayer life.

___
___
___
___

### DECIDE:
Consider the practical decisions you must make regarding this devotional. Write down those decisions and seek someone to keep you accountable.

___
___
___
___

### SURVEY:
Take note of your progress regarding this devotional. Changes don't happen suddenly but subtly. Write down any subtle improvements you notice over some time.

___
___
___
___

FATIGUE

## TOP THREE REASONS
## FOR WORKPLACE BURNOUT

*"The wages you failed to pay the workmen who mowed your fields are crying out against you. The cries of the harvesters have reached the ears of the Lord Almighty." James 5:4.*

According to a comprehensive study conducted by the World Health Organization (Michel, 2016), the top three reasons for burnout in the workplace are as follows. First, high job demands - unreasonable expectations from supervisors plunder your stamina. Second, low control - lacking the assets, ability, and authority to execute assignments deplete your motivation. Third, effort-reward imbalance - not being fairly compensated for your labor drain your vigor. Dr. Herbet Freudenberger was the first in behavioral science to coin the term "burnout" after investigating the climate of a New York City clinic in the 1970s, where each of the reasons above was a reality. He observed weariness, stress, and a growing cynicism towards the cliental amongst fatigued workers.

Recent studies in neuroscience confirm unprecedented changes in the brains of the burnt-out whereby cognitive skills and Amygdala are compromised (Hafeez, 2015). When burnout, bad decisions are easily made from a thinning of the prefrontal cortex. Emotional regulation becomes more complicated from an enlargement of the Amygdala that over-activates stress responses. Peruse through the stories of moral failure in the bible, and you'll see the evidence. For instance, Esau sells his birthright, Samson shares his secrets with Delilah, and David sins with Bathsheba, all at moments of tiredness to perhaps exhaustion. In each case, logical faculties failed while fleeting emotions prevailed.

If you're working under high demands, low control with inadequate compensation, you have an advocate with your Father in heaven. In James 5:4, the Apostle declares that God has heard the cries of those treated unjustly within the workplace. Take note, the scripture offers no assurance that your supervisors will hear your cries; facts are, some administrators are so elevated in attitude and altitude that they've lost touch with those at the bottom. Conversely, we have a God who hasn't lost his stoop. Psalm 138:6 tells us, "He sits up high but looks down low". If your complaints haven't been legitimatized by your employers, know that those complaints are recognized by your Savior. Anticipate divine intervention on your behalf as you cry out to Him.

---

### Related Verses:
*Galatians 6:9, Matthew 11:28-30, Genesis 25:29-34*

# DAILY M.E.D.S.:

*Apply this tool to receive the medicinal benefits of the devotional from the previous page.*

## MEDITATE:
Reflect upon the content of this devotional. Write, recite and mull over the key verses repeatedly until they reach your heart.

_____
_____
_____
_____

## ENGAGE:
Discuss this devotional with a trusted spiritual friend, pastor or counselor. Share your struggles relating to this devotional. Write whatever significant feedback they offer you. Most importantly, incorporate this devotional into your prayer life.

_____
_____
_____
_____

## DECIDE:
Consider the practical decisions you must make regarding this devotional. Write down those decisions and seek someone to keep you accountable.

_____
_____
_____
_____

## SURVEY:
Take note of your progress regarding this devotional. Changes don't happen suddenly but subtly. Write down any subtle improvements you notice over some time.

_____
_____
_____
_____

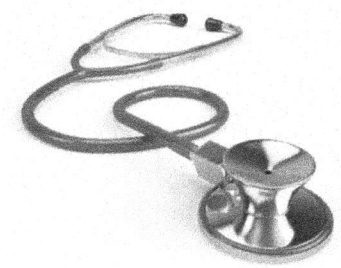

# GENERATIONAL CURSE:

*A predisposition towards certain dysfunctions
inherited from ancestors.*

<u>RELEVANT BIBLICAL PERSONALITIES:</u>
Manasseh (II Kings 21:3)
Amnon (II Kings 21:20)
Religious Leaders (John 8:39-47)
Jacob (Genesis 12:17, Genesis 27)

## ESCAPING YOUR PARENT'S SHADOWS

*"So Gideon went with ten men who were his servants and did just what the LORD had told him to do, though he did it at night because he was too afraid of his father's family and the leading men of the city to do it during the day." Judges 6:27*

Peculiarities are handed down from one generation to another through two mediums – what you were Taught and what you Caught. What you were Taught denotes not just what your parents said but how they behaved within your company. Isn't it amusing that we fuss about our kids not listening to us when we ought to worry that they are always watching us? For instance, adults who witnessed domestic violence when they were kids are 3-4 times more likely to perpetrate violence on their partners. Indeed, persuasive teachers leave an indelible mark on a pupil - not through their lectures - but lifestyles.

What you Caught refers to the more sophisticated transmission of genetics through the bloodline, a science we've barely scratched the surface in uncovering. Genetic transmissions are so bona fide that scientists verified twin siblings separated at birth possessed many similar behaviors in their adulthood, such as body postures and even religious persuasions (Bouchard, 1979). However, the study of Epigenetics reveals that you play an active role in choosing what genes to unlock. Life's great challenge is stepping into the divine light of who you are by crawling out of your parent's murky shadows.

In Judges 6, under the commands of Yahweh, Gideon demolishes his father's pagan-altars. For us, this act signifies breaking our ancestral shackles of alcoholism, sexual perversions, mental illnesses, etc. But, Gideon doesn't make such a bodacious move without caution and a militia. Gideon's decision to do it "by night" is the type of trepidation that's not fearful but careful (Not all fear is irrational). Furthermore, his choice to surround himself with a militia is wise. Every man/woman must be surrounded by a godly militia if he/she expects to break ties with an unholy tribe.

---

### Related Verses:
*II Corinthians 5:17, Psalm 79:8, Jeremiah 31:30*

Dr. JESUS

# DAILY M.E.D.S.:
*Apply this tool to receive the medicinal benefits of the devotional from the previous page.*

## MEDITATE:
Reflect upon the content of this devotional. Write, recite and mull over the key verses repeatedly until they reach your heart.

_____
_____
_____
_____

## ENGAGE:
Discuss this devotional with a trusted spiritual friend, pastor or counselor. Share your struggles relating to this devotional. Write whatever significant feedback they offer you. Most importantly, incorporate this devotional into your prayer life.

_____
_____
_____
_____

## DECIDE:
Consider the practical decisions you must make regarding this devotional. Write down those decisions and seek someone to keep you accountable.

_____
_____
_____
_____

## SURVEY:
Take note of your progress regarding this devotional. Changes don't happen suddenly but subtly. Write down any subtle improvements you notice over some time.

_____
_____
_____

# FREE-WILL TRUMPS GENETICS

*"Put away the gods that your fathers served beyond the River and in Egypt, and serve the Lord." Joshua 24:14*

No question that genetics are as persuasive as chocolate on a lonely night. The power of genetics is evident in the story of twins Jim Lewis & Jim Springer, who were separated from one another at four weeks old. When the two Jims reconciled in 1979, they discovered that they both smoked Salem cigarettes, bit their nails down to stubs, drove identical cars, and frequented the same locale at a Florida beach. Yet, they never met once in 39 years. Incontrovertibly, the 'gods your fathers served' were programmed from birth to be your default option at every decision point in life. Alcoholism, racism, personal preferences, and many predispositions are not just learned but burned into your hardwiring from the womb.

Before you surrender, know that genes have two functions. First, the TEMPLATE function is a biological software that determines how you look, prefer, and survive in particular environments. You have no control over the template function since it's inherited. Second, the TRANSCRIPTION function describes the turning-on of specific genes, and how those genes transcribe information upon your cells, rewiring your biology on a minute-by-minute basis based on choices. You have much say-so over this function based on your habitual decisions. Genes don't just shape you, but you most certainty shape them.

Without any understanding of genomics (the study of genes), Joshua knew thousands of years ago under the unction of God that we have the power to "put away" our father's idols. While every machine has a default function, it typically has a button called "settings," whereby you, the owner, have the prerogative to alter its default commands. Genetics may have some say, but they do not have the final say in the outcome of your life. The person you become will not be merely the result of your dispositions but the outcome of your decisions. Choose rightly.

---

### Related Verses:
*Joshua 24:14-15, Deuteronomy 30:15-20, John 10:10*

Dr. JESUS

# DAILY M.E.D.S.:
*Apply this tool to receive the medicinal benefits of the devotional from the previous page.*

## MEDITATE:
Reflect upon the content of this devotional. Write, recite and mull over the key verses repeatedly until they reach your heart.

_____
_____
_____
_____

## ENGAGE:
Discuss this devotional with a trusted spiritual friend, pastor or counselor. Share your struggles relating to this devotional. Write whatever significant feedback they offer you. Most importantly, incorporate this devotional into your prayer life.

_____
_____
_____
_____

## DECIDE:
Consider the practical decisions you must make regarding this devotional. Write down those decisions and seek someone to keep you accountable.

_____
_____
_____
_____

## SURVEY:
Take note of your progress regarding this devotional. Changes don't happen suddenly but subtly. Write down any subtle improvements you notice over some time.

_____
_____
_____
_____

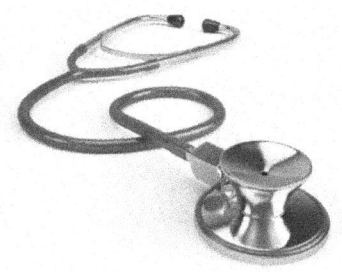

# GRIEF:

*An intense emotional and physical reaction followed by the loss of someone or something that manifests a variety of emotions such as sadness, anger, denial and bargaining.*

RELEVANT BIBLICAL PERSONALITIES:
Jesus (John 11:35)
Jacob (Genesis 37:24)
David (II Samuel 12:13-25)
Job (Job 2:13)
Jairus' family (Mark 5:38)
Martha & Mary (John 11)

# "I'M OVER IT"

*"Blessed are those who mourn, for they shall be comforted." Matthew 5:4.*

I once injured my shin during a morning workout routine without even knowing it. Injury awareness occurred many hours later when a throbbing sensation shot across my leg as if I'd been bit by a shark. Why such a delay? Endorphins are hormones secreted within the nervous system, released during stressful moments, that alleviate pain. Endorphins are often dubbed by doctors "the natural opiates of the body", tricking the mind into thinking all is well even when you're going through hell. Here's the kick in the head - Endorphins are also activated during life crises, such as losing a loved one, abandonment, divorce, being fired, etc. Endorphins make you think, "I'm over it", when you haven't even begun! (Hence, the reason why the very first stage of grief is known as DENIAL).

Truly getting "over" something traumatic only occurs after you traverse through the tunnel of grief. Grief is likened to a tunnel because the only way to reach its terminus is to go through it. You can't get through grief without actually grieving. There's no way around it! Back in the 1960s, Dr. Elizabeth Kubler-Ross studied innumerable patients who grieved terminally ill loved ones. From her data analysis, she constructed the "Five Stages of Grief Model" which includes Denial, Anger, Bargaining, Depression, and Acceptance. Permitting yourself the freedom to experience all five emotions while processing your support system is the only way through the tunnel of grief. The final stage, Acceptance, includes cortisol regulation (which means not feeling stressed by previously traumatizing events).

Almost 2,000 years before the Kubler-Ross model, Dr. Jesus uttered a simple statement that speaks vividly about getting over loss in Matthew 5:4. The Greek term for "Mourn" means "manifesting your grief over any loss whatsoever." The term highlights our inherent need to express sorrow to make our way out of it. You'll notice the practice of mourning throughout the bible as men and women experience losses of any kind. All this to say, if you've indeed reached the end of the tunnel, you should be able to look back and see a passageway of darkness. Dawn doesn't arrive until hours of evening pass by. If not, the endorphins may not have even subsided yet. Are you really "over it"?

---

### Related Verses:
*John 11:35, James 4:9, Psalm 126:5*

Dr. JESUS

# DAILY M.E.D.S.:
*Apply this tool to receive the medicinal benefits of the devotional from the previous page.*

## MEDITATE:
Reflect upon the content of this devotional. Write, recite and mull over the key verses repeatedly until they reach your heart.

___
___
___
___

## ENGAGE:
Discuss this devotional with a trusted spiritual friend, pastor or counselor. Share your struggles relating to this devotional. Write whatever significant feedback they offer you. Most importantly, incorporate this devotional into your prayer life.

___
___
___
___

## DECIDE:
Consider the practical decisions you must make regarding this devotional. Write down those decisions and seek someone to keep you accountable.

___
___
___
___

## SURVEY:
Take note of your progress regarding this devotional. Changes don't happen suddenly but subtly. Write down any subtle improvements you notice over some time.

___
___
___
___

# GRIEF AND FAMILY DYNAMICS
*"Martha went out to find Jesus while Mary stayed home." John 11:20.*

80-90% of married couples that lost a child will divorce within a few years after the tragedy (Rando, 1985). Many families stop nestling around the dinner table or practicing long-held customs after bereaving any cherished relative. The recipes are forgotten, the photo albums buried in a musty basement, and stories of the homeland become hazy. Tribes scatter rather than gather for many reasons - one reason being clashing expressions of grief.

In Eric Clapton's interview with Larry King, he shed light on the ultra-sensitivity between him and his partner after their 4-year-old son, Conor, fell to his death from an open apartment window in Manhattan. Clapton spoke about how introverted he became in his grief while Lori was demonstrative. He rationalized their grieving differences as cultural (English being reserved while Italians being passionate) but couldn't minimize the awful effects on his relationship. Clapton implicitly alluded to the diverse ways we express sorrow based on personality traits, religions, and cultural differences. We are ignorant in presuming our way of grieving is the golden standard.

It is fascinating to note Martha and Mary's contrasting reactions to the death of their beloved brother, Lazarus. Martha hits the streets looking for Jesus to change what's been done, while Mary remains in the house of mourners accepting the grim reality. According to the studies of Martin & Dakota, there are two common grief languages - Instrumental Grievers and Intuitive Grievers. Instrumental Grievers (Martha) channel their sorrow through activities inspired by the loss of their loved one. Intuitive Grievers (Mary) go inward, expressing their sorrow through pensive thoughts and profound affect. Martin & Dakota's research call for the grieving individual to express their sorrow authentically. But also, for the sake of family preservation, a call is made to respect the differences of others. One of the most important truths we can remember when grieving amongst others is that different doesn't mean deficient. Let it be understood that Martha and Mary are both doting siblings.

---

**Related Verses:**
*Philippians 2:3, Matthew 7:12, II Corinthians 1:3-4*

# DAILY M.E.D.S.:

*Apply this tool to receive the medicinal benefits of the devotional from the previous page.*

## MEDITATE:
Reflect upon the content of this devotional. Write, recite and mull over the key verses repeatedly until they reach your heart.

_____
_____
_____
_____

## ENGAGE:
Discuss this devotional with a trusted spiritual friend, pastor or counselor. Share your struggles relating to this devotional. Write whatever significant feedback they offer you. Most importantly, incorporate this devotional into your prayer life.

_____
_____
_____
_____

## DECIDE:
Consider the practical decisions you must make regarding this devotional. Write down those decisions and seek someone to keep you accountable.

_____
_____
_____
_____

## SURVEY:
Take note of your progress regarding this devotional. Changes don't happen suddenly but subtly. Write down any subtle improvements you notice over some time.

_____
_____
_____
_____

# WHO SAYS YOU SHOULDN'T BE SAD! DISENFRANCHISED GRIEF

*"Jesus wept." John 11:35.*

I slit my infected finger with a sanitized blade, permitting the greenish pus to ooze out from the incision. Oftentimes, healing doesn't occur without hurting. Cutting myself, in this particular context, is an act of service to my body. The cut reminded me of Hamlet's words in that legendary Shakespeare play, "I must be cruel to be kind". Similarly, mourning is an act of service to the soul, an expression of self-care after enduring loss. Albeit mourning might be as agonizing as slitting my finger, such rendering of the soul allows the pus of anger, bitterness and other melancholy emotions to ooze out.

Disenfranchised grief is the inability to mourn because of certain social pressures that forbid you to do so. For instance, a Christian teenager conceives a child out of wedlock. Soon after, she miscarries. She's expected to be happy given the fact that the baby was born "in sin". She swallows her tears rather than shedding them; hence, she becomes severely depressed. Or how about the woman not expected to grieve her father's passing since he molested her, or the man not allowed to mourn the loss of a marriage since it was dysfunctional anyway. Family and friends describe such losses as "blessings in disguise", yet these losses leave its victims in a quiet desperation of the soul.

Jesus wept. Nobody expects him to weep. He is the Savior of the world with supernatural power in his hands to raise Lazarus from the dead. Yet still, He cries like a baby. Even he himself could rationalize away his hurt by thinking, "Lazarus is just a few minutes away from returning to life!". Yet still, he soaks the rug beneath his feet. When the entire world forbids you from weeping, Jesus hands you a box of tissue.

---

### Related Verses:
*Psalms 126:5-6, II Samuel 12:16-23, Psalm 34:18, Proverbs 14:13*

# DAILY M.E.D.S.:
*Apply this tool to receive the medicinal benefits of the devotional from the previous page.*

## MEDITATE:
Reflect upon the content of this devotional. Write, recite and mull over the key verses repeatedly until they reach your heart.

_____
_____
_____
_____

## ENGAGE:
Discuss this devotional with a trusted spiritual friend, pastor or counselor. Share your struggles relating to this devotional. Write whatever significant feedback they offer you. Most importantly, incorporate this devotional into your prayer life.

_____
_____
_____
_____

## DECIDE:
Consider the practical decisions you must make regarding this devotional. Write down those decisions and seek someone to keep you accountable.

_____
_____
_____
_____

## SURVEY:
Take note of your progress regarding this devotional. Changes don't happen suddenly but subtly. Write down any subtle improvements you notice over some time.

_____
_____
_____
_____

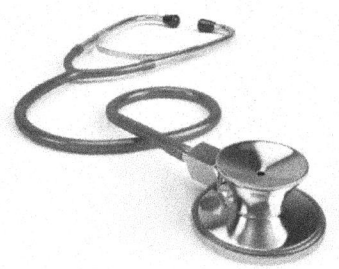

# HOARDING:

*Persistent difficulty discarding or parting with possessions because of a perceived need to save them.*

RELEVANT BIBLICAL PERSONALITIES:
Rich Young Ruler (Mark 10:17-27)
Rich Man (Luke 16:19-31)
Judas (John 12:6)
Wealthy land-owners (James 5:4)

# WHEN POSSESSIONS POSSESS US

*"Jesus said to the rich young ruler, 'Sell your possessions and bless the poor.'" Luke 18:22.*

We all have a hoarding instinct, a cemented grip on the stuff we cherish. Remember your reaction to that fool in the nursery who swiped your doll - you bopped them between the eyes with it. "Mine!" was perhaps the earliest term you uttered as instinctively as belching. Ironically, minutes after you reclaimed your doll from that little creep's hands, you tossed it aside to play with the big round ball.

But why such a tight grip? Indeed, you don't cherish your stuff for practical purposes alone. If that were the case, President John F. Kennedy's tape measure wouldn't auction for $48,475 when one could be purchased for $1.07 at the Dollar Tree. 93% of Americans wouldn't own running shoes when only a handful run, and people wouldn't own so many books that they don't even read.

What makes stuff so powerful is not what it does for us but what it says about us (to our fragile egos and attentive peers). Owning JFK's tape-measure makes the brassy statement, "I'm special!" the running shoes proudly say, "I'm fit!" and the books boast, "I'm smart!". We cherish our stuff, not because it brings us utility, but because it boosts our identity.

In other dialogues w aristocrats, Jesus issues no such command to rid possessions. Yet, with this man, Jesus tells him to relinquish it all. This man possibly foolishly sought something from his stuff that it wasn't designed to give him, such as a boost of identity. A study conducted at Knox College (Deangelis, 2004) indicated that the more people esteemed their possessions, the higher they scored for depression. Possessions make terrific toys but make horrific gods. Only Jesus himself could reach down that deep within you.

---

### Related Verses:
*Matthew 6:19-24, Luke 16:19-31, II Corinthians 1:3-4*

# DAILY M.E.D.S.:

*Apply this tool to receive the medicinal benefits of the devotional from the previous page.*

### MEDITATE:
Reflect upon the content of this devotional. Write, recite and mull over the key verses repeatedly until they reach your heart.

_____
_____
_____
_____

### ENGAGE:
Discuss this devotional with a trusted spiritual friend, pastor or counselor. Share your struggles relating to this devotional. Write whatever significant feedback they offer you. Most importantly, incorporate this devotional into your prayer life.

_____
_____
_____
_____

### DECIDE:
Consider the practical decisions you must make regarding this devotional. Write down those decisions and seek someone to keep you accountable.

_____
_____
_____
_____

### SURVEY:
Take note of your progress regarding this devotional. Changes don't happen suddenly but subtly. Write down any subtle improvements you notice over some time.

_____
_____
_____
_____

# WORTHLESS ATTACHMENTS

*"Do not store up for yourselves treasures on earth where moths and vermin destroy and where thieves break in and steal. But store up for yourselves treasures in heaven, where moths and vermin do not destroy, and where thieves do not break in and steal." Matthew 6:19-20.*

Next time your hosting company (let's say, four people), gift two mugs from your cabinet to half your company. Ask the two people who were gifted the mugs to tell you the lowest price they would sell it for. Ask the other two folks to tell you the highest price they would pay for the mug. Chances are, the mug owner's minimum selling price is 2-3 x the amount of the other folk's buying price. The Endowment Effect is an emotional bias whereby we place on something a higher value than what it's worth simply because it belongs to us (Kahneman, 1991). The instant we forge an attachment with anything, it becomes priceless within our fantastical minds even when it's worthless. For instance, you might hear someone say....

"Meet MY boyfriend. Yes, I know he left his fist print under my eye and fools around w/ my girlfriend. But he's MY boyfriend!"

"Let me tell you about MY grudge against mom and dad. Yes, I know that the grudge has transfigured me into a bitter, unloveable man. But, it's MY grudge."

"Let me show you MY bank statement. Yes, I know these assets split my family apart in more ways than one. But these are MY assets!"

Under such a spell, we place a high price on stuff that offers us a low life. In Matthew 6, Jesus alludes to this effect. He expounds upon how we "treasure" stuff that disappoints us in the final analysis. Jesus then offers us a remedy for such insanity. Set your affections on heaven while living on this side of eternity. Win souls, develop meaningful relationships, take care of the poor, etc. By doing these things, you invest in the only asset (Jesus himself) that offers eternal perpetuity.

---

## Related Verses:
*Colossians 3:2, Matthew 25:40-45, Matthew 6:33*

Dr. JESUS

# DAILY M.E.D.S.:
*Apply this tool to receive the medicinal benefits of the devotional from the previous page.*

## MEDITATE:
Reflect upon the content of this devotional. Write, recite and mull over the key verses repeatedly until they reach your heart.

_____
_____
_____
_____

## ENGAGE:
Discuss this devotional with a trusted spiritual friend, pastor or counselor. Share your struggles relating to this devotional. Write whatever significant feedback they offer you. Most importantly, incorporate this devotional into your prayer life.

_____
_____
_____
_____

## DECIDE:
Consider the practical decisions you must make regarding this devotional. Write down those decisions and seek someone to keep you accountable.

_____
_____
_____
_____

## SURVEY:
Take note of your progress regarding this devotional. Changes don't happen suddenly but subtly. Write down any subtle improvements you notice over some time.

_____
_____
_____
_____

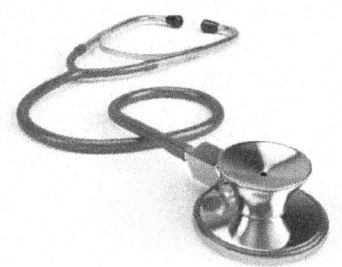

# INSECURITY:

*A feeling of inadequacy, lack of confidence and the inability to cope.*

<u>RELEVANT BIBLICAL PERSONALITIES:</u>
Cain (Genesis 4)
Saul (I Samuel 10:22)
Elkanah (I Samuel 1:8)
Timothy (II Timothy 1:7)
Moses (Exodus 4:10-13)

## YOU DON'T KNOW A THING ABOUT ME

*"Eliab, David's oldest brother, said to him, 'Why have you come down here?....I know how conceited you are and how wicked your heart is; you came down only to watch the battle.'" I Samuel 17*

Decades ago in a French town, residents hosted a Charlie Chaplin look-a-like contest. Chaplin fanatics voted on the dude who resembled their beloved actor the most. Unbeknownst to the town residents, the real Chaplin slipped into the contest and was voted on. The funny thing is, the real Charlie Chaplin came in 3rd!....Don't take to heart what people claim to see in you, even those who supposedly know you best, because many factors grossly impair their perspective. You could accurately recite the words of Kelly Clarkson to some of your closest peeps, "You don't know a thing about me".

A leading reason why folk's opinions of you are compromised is Projection. Sigmund Freud conceptualized the Theory of Projection after realizing an interplay between a patient's shame and views of their neighbors as gossipy and evil. Freud observed a pattern whereby his patient deflected attention away from self-awareness by talking about the neighbor's cruel ways. From this incident, Freud conjured that we project our defects towards other people to avoid looking at ourselves. Rather than addressing his hang-ups, the patient turned critical towards his neighbors. When I project, I lay into you so that I don't have to look at myself. For this reason, people's opinions of you are not always trustworthy; sometimes, they turn you into the whipping post for their own defects.

In our focal passage, David's older brother accuses him of being conceited. Such a harsh, unfair judgment at a moment when David delivers a sandwich to his brother on the battlefield! David is called conceited in the same instant that he shows himself to be considerate. From what data does the brother formulate such a judgment? Perhaps David's brother is arrogant since he's the one out front ready to kill Goliath for all the townspeople to see. Some people spot what they got; acute projection rather than keen perception. Fortunately, David's heart is inclined to care more about what God thinks than what his brother supposes. If you've been taking to heart what other people say about you, please know that the only applause that matters is from nail-scarred hands. Your critics should go pound sand in Jesus' name.

---

### Related Verses:
*Galatians 1:10, I Samuel 16:7, Proverbs 20:5*

# DAILY M.E.D.S.:

*Apply this tool to receive the medicinal benefits of the devotional from the previous page.*

## MEDITATE:
Reflect upon the content of this devotional. Write, recite and mull over the key verses repeatedly until they reach your heart.

_____
_____
_____
_____

## ENGAGE:
Discuss this devotional with a trusted spiritual friend, pastor or counselor. Share your struggles relating to this devotional. Write whatever significant feedback they offer you. Most importantly, incorporate this devotional into your prayer life.

_____
_____
_____
_____

## DECIDE:
Consider the practical decisions you must make regarding this devotional. Write down those decisions and seek someone to keep you accountable.

_____
_____
_____
_____

## SURVEY:
Take note of your progress regarding this devotional. Changes don't happen suddenly but subtly. Write down any subtle improvements you notice over some time.

_____
_____
_____
_____

## SHATTERING STIGMA
*"Jesus saw a certain widow..." Luke 21:2*

"You shocked me with how smart you are", she spewed after hearing me lecture on social influences, not so carefully concealing her hoity-toity outlook. What did you expect of me? Slick black hair, Mediterranean complexion with a thick Italo-American brogue, perhaps you presumed I'd be dicing garlic in a Federal Hill eatery or breaking knees for the local crime family. Such nerve of a fellow like me carrying on within the collegiate setting! After all these years of higher education (B.A., M.Ed., Ph.D.), you'd think by now I'd shed the usage of urban colloquialisms, clean up my diction and dress more Oxfords. I get it. I don't look the part. I still act very much "Italian," yakking with a mouth full of ravioli, motioning like a mime when making a point, and sounding like I swallowed a microphone at three years old. I don't seem to fit in the world of academia.

Living under stigma is no easy thing. I can't imagine what ladies feel like in a boardroom supervised by men. "Women are emotional beings, devoid of logic," says one fellow. There are so many stigmas surrounding the mentally ill, the physically disabled, the financially impoverished, and a host of other ethnic stereotypes that make the journey challenging. You grossly underestimate our social nature if you think it's a simple thing to shrug off stigmas. Word, Zanna, and Cooper (1974) demonstrated within an experiment that African Americans poorly performed when interviewed by managers who made implicitly prejudiced gestures compared to applicants treated justly. Being stigmatized rocks us to the core.

In bible days, widows had a reputation for being "on the take." Living without a husband in a patriarchal society turned you into a ward of society. In our era, we might call them a "welfare case." When she made her way into the temple, I'm sure the religious leaders were thinking, "Here comes another widow! Just another leech!". But in Luke 21:2, the bible doesn't say, "Jesus saw just another widow"; instead, it says, "Jesus saw a CERTAIN widow." The term, CERTAIN, means that Jesus perceived the particularities of this woman's personality, not according to her social class or stigma. This certain widow didn't look the part! She came giving rather than taking, and Jesus recognized her for who she was. All this to say, overcoming stigma begins with seeing yourself in the vivid reflection of Jesus' eyes rather than the murky feedback of ignoramuses. Sometimes, people don't know a thing about you, but Jesus does.

### Related Verses:
*James 2:1-26, Matthew 7:1-5, John 7:24*

# DAILY M.E.D.S.:

*Apply this tool to receive the medicinal benefits of the devotional from the previous page.*

## MEDITATE:
Reflect upon the content of this devotional. Write, recite and mull over the key verses repeatedly until they reach your heart.

_____
_____
_____
_____

## ENGAGE:
Discuss this devotional with a trusted spiritual friend, pastor or counselor. Share your struggles relating to this devotional. Write whatever significant feedback they offer you. Most importantly, incorporate this devotional into your prayer life.

_____
_____
_____
_____

## DECIDE:
Consider the practical decisions you must make regarding this devotional. Write down those decisions and seek someone to keep you accountable.

_____
_____
_____
_____

## SURVEY:
Take note of your progress regarding this devotional. Changes don't happen suddenly but subtly. Write down any subtle improvements you notice over some time.

_____
_____
_____
_____

# THE MIDLIFE CRISIS
*"All is vanity!" Ecclesiastes 1:2*

A Midlife Crisis is more than mythical, but a reality that bites hard for a large percentage of people between the ages of 40-55 years old. A national survey conducted by Very Well Mind (Cherry, 2020) indicated that 26% of people at midlife undergo an emotional crisis consisting of one or more of the quintessential characteristics – extramarital affairs, substantial financial purchases, drastic plastic surgery, and a host of other impulsive decisions. This begs the question, What are the underlying factors of a Midlife Crisis?

Existential grief is the prelude to almost every Midlife Crisis. Existential grief is a spell of meaninglessness cast upon the minds of men and women, typically between the ages of 40-60 years old. Folks who suffer from existential grief lose touch with the reason behind all their routines, forgetting the "Why" behind whatever they do. Under this melancholy enchantment, all of life appears as pointless as "chasing the wind." King Solomon, a man so wealthy that archeologists are still uncovering his assets thousands of years later, surveys all that he owns and says, "Vanity!". The king's confessions parallel the words of Muhammad Ali, who told a reporter, "I had the world, and it ain't nuttin."

If you've been hexed with existential grief, put the brakes on your decisions. Why? Allow me to answer with a story. Once upon a time, a young man cut down an oversized tree on a frigid January day. A few months later, he walked through the woods with his father & noticed new shoots sprouting around the trunk. "I thought for sure it was dead when I cut it down," the young man said to his father. The wise father replied, "Let this be a lesson to you. Never cut down a tree on a cold winter day. Never make a drastic decision at a low point in your life. What appears dead may have more vitality within its roots than what your eyes perceive. God forbid you should put an end to something so valuable."

---

## Related Verses:
*James 4:14, Psalm 90:12-17, Proverbs 4:26*

# DAILY M.E.D.S.:
*Apply this tool to receive the medicinal benefits of the devotional from the previous page.*

## MEDITATE:
Reflect upon the content of this devotional. Write, recite and mull over the key verses repeatedly until they reach your heart.

_____
_____
_____
_____

## ENGAGE:
Discuss this devotional with a trusted spiritual friend, pastor or counselor. Share your struggles relating to this devotional. Write whatever significant feedback they offer you. Most importantly, incorporate this devotional into your prayer life.

_____
_____
_____
_____

## DECIDE:
Consider the practical decisions you must make regarding this devotional. Write down those decisions and seek someone to keep you accountable.

_____
_____
_____
_____

## SURVEY:
Take note of your progress regarding this devotional. Changes don't happen suddenly but subtly. Write down any subtle improvements you notice over some time.

_____
_____
_____
_____

## REASONS WHY YOU SHOULD EMBRACE BEING A MISFIT

*"I am a foreigner in a foreign land." Exodus 2:22.*

Moses was too Egyptian to fit in with the Hebrews yet too Hebrew to fit in with the Egyptians. No matter where he dwelt, he felt like an outsider within that particular terrain. Hence, the reason he says, "I am a foreigner in this land!". Paul was too Jewish to fit in with the early Christians, yet too Christian to fit in with the Jews (I use these descriptors loosely). Paul and Moses were misfits. Are you a misfit? If you find yourself standing out rather than fitting in, here are a few reasons to embrace your status.

1. OBJECTIVITY - A handful of engineers detected faulty mechanical issues in building the Challenger Space Shuttle but suppressed their findings to conform to their peers. Passion to launch the space shuttle was the consensus, so those engineers went along to get along (a phenomenon known as, Group-Think). Sadly, seven people were killed 73 seconds after its launch as the Challenger exploded on January 28, 1986. Countless studies show that the more we try to fit in with the group, the more we suppress innovative ideas and keen observational skills. Conversely, folks secure with being on the fringes possess an objective viewpoint that insiders often lack.

2. EMPATHY - Cheung and Gardner (2014) performed a study amongst 101 online pen-pal writing group participants. Findings indicated that the most socially excluded within the group demonstrated the highest levels of empathy to pen-pals who recently experienced loss. Being a misfit tenderizes your heart, enabling you to perceive the world through the teary eyes of others.

3. INTIMACY - Relationships are established upon the common ground; hence, the reason for the prefix, Relate. You cannot have a relationship with whom you cannot relate. Being a misfit allows us to deepen our bond with Jesus. He, himself, is the ultimate misfit, too heavenly to fit in on earth, yet the only one in heaven who walked this earth. Moments of social exclusion are opportunities for misfits to find a friend in Jesus Christ who chooses rejects to be His closest confidants (I Corinthians 1:26).

---

### Related Verses:
*I Corinthians 1:26, Psalm 138:6, Ecclesiastes 7:13*

# DAILY M.E.D.S.:

*Apply this tool to receive the medicinal benefits of the devotional from the previous page.*

### MEDITATE:
Reflect upon the content of this devotional. Write, recite and mull over the key verses repeatedly until they reach your heart.

_____
_____
_____
_____

### ENGAGE:
Discuss this devotional with a trusted spiritual friend, pastor or counselor. Share your struggles relating to this devotional. Write whatever significant feedback they offer you. Most importantly, incorporate this devotional into your prayer life.

_____
_____
_____
_____

### DECIDE:
Consider the practical decisions you must make regarding this devotional. Write down those decisions and seek someone to keep you accountable.

_____
_____
_____
_____

### SURVEY:
Take note of your progress regarding this devotional. Changes don't happen suddenly but subtly. Write down any subtle improvements you notice over some time.

_____
_____
_____
_____

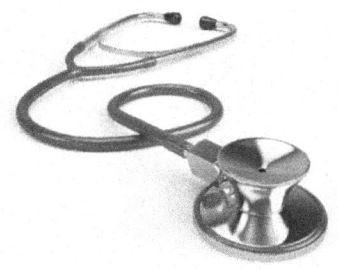

# NARCISSISM:

*An inordinate interest or preoccupation with oneself
along with entitlement, arrogance and the exploitation of others.*

<u>Relevant Biblical personalities:</u>
Herod (Matthew 2:1-12)
Pharaoh (Exodus 5)
Eve (Genesis 3:5)
Saul (I Samuel 15:30)

# WHAT IS HUMILITY?

*"When you've been invited to a banquet, seat yourself in the lowest place. When the guest of honor arrives, he will say to you, 'Friend, come up higher.'" Luke 14:7-11*

What makes a person humble? Recent studies in behavioral science show that the most common characteristic amongst people who scored high on a humility questionnaire was NOT downplaying one's accomplishments or positive traits, such as when people deny their gifts when complimented. That kind of humility is as superficial and dishonest as Botox. Instead, the hallmark of humility was indicated as being "hypo-egoic non-entitlement"; a fancy way of saying that you don't believe your positive traits or accolades qualify you for special treatment (Leary, 2004). The truly humble person finds their seat amongst the beggars even if they hold a royal pedigree. This attitude flies in the face of the narcissistic impulse to elevate oneself in the sight of people.

When literary Thomas Hardy was so famous that any London newspaper would have gladly paid him mega-bucks for his writings, he submitted his poems to local editors with a stamped envelope inside every package. Why? Just in case the newspaper rejected his work, the editor could mail him back his poems. Hardy was a humble man who didn't presume his fame guaranteed him a spot in the sun. Hypo-egoic entitlement means that you know you're gifted, but don't assume your gifts entitle you to rose petals and red carpets.

In Luke 14, Jesus divulges the counterintuitive rewards of being humble. If a man seats himself amongst the common folk at a banquet, that same man shall be granted the privilege of sitting front and center. He receives the very thing he didn't demand. Honor falls upon the humble, and special treatment is extended to those who don't insist upon it.

---

### Related Verses:
*Philippians 2:5-11, James 4:10, Matthew 5:3*

# DAILY M.E.D.S.:

*Apply this tool to receive the medicinal benefits of the devotional from the previous page.*

## MEDITATE:
Reflect upon the content of this devotional. Write, recite and mull over the key verses repeatedly until they reach your heart.

_____
_____
_____
_____

## ENGAGE:
Discuss this devotional with a trusted spiritual friend, pastor or counselor. Share your struggles relating to this devotional. Write whatever significant feedback they offer you. Most importantly, incorporate this devotional into your prayer life.

_____
_____
_____
_____

## DECIDE:
Consider the practical decisions you must make regarding this devotional. Write down those decisions and seek someone to keep you accountable.

_____
_____
_____
_____

## SURVEY:
Take note of your progress regarding this devotional. Changes don't happen suddenly but subtly. Write down any subtle improvements you notice over some time.

_____
_____
_____
_____

## WHAT LIES BEHIND NARCISSISM?

*"Look," Pharaoh said to his people, "the Israelites have become far too numerous for us." Exodus 1:9*

Behind every superiority complex, deep-seated inferiority plagues the soul. In his 229-page report, "Analysis of the Personality of Adolph Hitler" (1943), Harvard professor Dr. Henry Murray conjectures that Hitler camouflaged before the masses a profound self-loathing that stemmed from being a frail, sickly child with severe academic handicaps. Recently, New York University conducted a survey amongst 300 participants on narcissism. The survey showed narcissism is not driven by a grandiose sense of self but just the opposite - a fragile psyche working hard to protect itself from seeing its own "despicable" reflection (Kowalchyk, 2020). As farmers say in the Deep South, "the Hen that crows the loudest lays the smallest eggs."

At some point in your life, you might be targeted by a narcissist - a bullying spouse, a browbeating supervisor, or a belittling sibling. Every chance they get to make you feel small is seized as swiftly as taking free money. Hanging around a Narcissist long enough can take its toll on your self-esteem. A sure indication you need space from such a person is when their harassing voice mutates into your thoughts about yourself. (If you suppose it's unchristian for me to talk this way, do yourself a favor by reading II Timothy 3:1-17 with particular attention to the phrase, "avoid such people"). If a narcissist has targeted you, you need to know what you're dealing with.

On the surface, Pharaoh is a maniacal tyrant scouting for an opportunity to flaunt his dominance over the defenseless Jews. Read through Exodus 5, and you'll encounter a Monster who gleans satisfaction from stomping upon the souls of God's people. But, behind the scenes, Pharaoh is petrified of the very people he oppresses. Exodus 1:9 allows us access to Pharaoh's intimate circle, where he utters his true feelings. Essentially, he says, "These people scare the wits out of me!" If a narcissist has browbeaten you, understand that you've been targeted, NOT because of how pathetic you are, but how intimidating your intellect, talent, virtue, or whatever else comes across to them. Be not afraid of the narcissist; at the heart of every bully is a baby.

---

### Related Verses:
*II Timothy 3:1-17, Romans 16:17-19, Exodus 5*

# DAILY M.E.D.S.:

*Apply this tool to receive the medicinal benefits of the devotional from the previous page.*

## MEDITATE:
Reflect upon the content of this devotional. Write, recite and mull over the key verses repeatedly until they reach your heart.

_____
_____
_____
_____

## ENGAGE:
Discuss this devotional with a trusted spiritual friend, pastor or counselor. Share your struggles relating to this devotional. Write whatever significant feedback they offer you. Most importantly, incorporate this devotional into your prayer life.

_____
_____
_____
_____

## DECIDE:
Consider the practical decisions you must make regarding this devotional. Write down those decisions and seek someone to keep you accountable.

_____
_____
_____
_____

## SURVEY:
Take note of your progress regarding this devotional. Changes don't happen suddenly but subtly. Write down any subtle improvements you notice over some time.

_____
_____
_____
_____

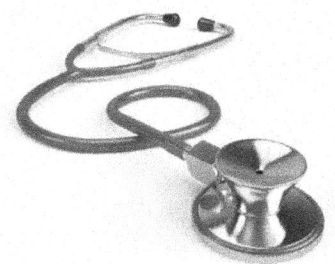

# OBSESSIVE COMPULSIVE DISORDER:

*A disorder in which people have recurring, unwanted thoughts, ideas or sensations (obsessions) that make them feel driven to do something repetitively (compulsions).*

RELEVANT BIBLICAL PERSONALITIES:
Paul (Romans 7)
The Pharisees (Matthew 23, Luke 11:39)

# ORIGINS OF OBSESSIVE-COMPULSIVE DISORDER (O.C.D.)

*"There is no fear in love. But perfect love drives out fear, because fear has to do with punishment." I John 4:18.*

'Push-ups' was a middle-aged man in our neighborhood who hit the pavement in mid-conversation to bang out a set of push-ups. At first glance, he practiced this ritual for no apparent reason other than being a health fanatic. But really, he was scared to death of not being physically equipped for an enemy that could strike at any hour (a fear he acquired in combat). O.C.D. behaviors are not merely the rituals of a fanatic but are rooted in deep fears. For instance, a woman doesn't just alphabetize her canned goods because she's a neat freak; in some cases, she's subconsciously scared of being punished by a tyrant parent. If you suffer with O.C.D., ask yourself, "What am I afraid of happening if I don't practice this ritual?"

In 1976, Roper & Rachman experimented on patients with O.C.D. They noted that all symptoms dissipated shortly after the patients were admitted into their labs. Researchers didn't know why symptoms disappeared until the patients left the lab to return to everyday life and their rituals returned with a fury. After further investigation, Roper & Rachman learned that the symptoms disappeared in the lab because the patients mentally transferred horrible outcomes of not practicing rituals to the researchers. The forethought of a bad outcome is what perpetuates O.C.D. rituals.

In our focal passage, the Apostle John brilliantly correlates the emotion of fear (the driving force behind O.C.D.) with impending punishment. This punishment-frightened thought process is a powerful impetus that causes someone to make sure every shirt is lined up, and every crumb vacuumed. The Apostle introduces the only cure for this torment – perfect love. Perfect love is a love that persists even when you're imperfect. Many years ago, an Olympic swimmer was asked if he was afraid of failure. He responded, "No because whether I make the drive or not, I know my mother still loves me." Fear cannot survive where love thrives.

---

### Related Verses:
*John 3:17, II Timothy 1:7, Isaiah 41:10*

Dr. JESUS

# DAILY M.E.D.S.:
*Apply this tool to receive the medicinal benefits of the devotional from the previous page.*

## MEDITATE:
Reflect upon the content of this devotional. Write, recite and mull over the key verses repeatedly until they reach your heart.

_____
_____
_____
_____

## ENGAGE:
Discuss this devotional with a trusted spiritual friend, pastor or counselor. Share your struggles relating to this devotional. Write whatever significant feedback they offer you. Most importantly, incorporate this devotional into your prayer life.

_____
_____
_____
_____

## DECIDE:
Consider the practical decisions you must make regarding this devotional. Write down those decisions and seek someone to keep you accountable.

_____
_____
_____
_____

## SURVEY:
Take note of your progress regarding this devotional. Changes don't happen suddenly but subtly. Write down any subtle improvements you notice over some time.

_____
_____
_____

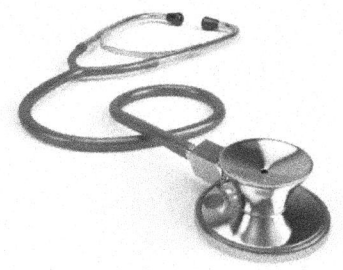

# PARANOIA:

*Anxious feelings relating to persecution, threat or conspiracies.*

### RELEVANT BIBLICAL PERSONALITIES:
Saul (I Samuel 22:8, 13-19)

Pharaoh & Egyptians (Exodus 1:12)

The Wicked (Proverbs 28:1)

Demoniac Man (Matthew 8:28)

# THE PSYCHOLOGY BEHIND CONSPIRACY THEORIES

*"Do not call conspiracy everything this people calls a conspiracy; do not fear what they fear." Isaiah 8:12*

Back in the 1980s, it was a view amongst bug-eyed folks that H.I.V. was a virus designed by the government to curtail population increase. When catastrophes erupt, some folks are predisposed to paranoia by believing conspiracy theories. Why do some folks buy into conspiracy theories? According to the prophet Isaiah, "fear" is the underlying issue of conspiracy theories. Lend me your ear....

Have you ever hung out in the company of people when a circumstance went wrong? For instance, you're driving in a remote town with a group of friends when your car breaks down. With the hood up, you over-hear your passengers chitchatting about why this happened. A few of your passengers understand that these things occur simply because that's the nature of life - pretty flowers wither, beautiful people age, and nice cars malfunction. Several other passengers seek an explanation where someone is at fault for what happened. They might even come up with a conspiracy theory on how Ford designs their cars to malfunction.

In this situation, two kinds of explanations surface amongst your passengers – situational attributions and dispositional attributions. A situational attribution is when we attribute what went wrong to living in an imperfect world. People that make situational attributions comprehend things go wrong simply because that's the nature of life. Dispositional attributions attribute what went wrong to the fault of a person(s); if something goes wrong, someone is to blame! People who make these attributions believe that the disposition of man (as evil, incompetent, etc.) is the reason behind every problem that occurs. At its core, a conspiracy theory is a dispositional attribution where a problem is being blamed on person(s), usually at the highest level.

How does all of this relate to "fear" (the reason behind conspiracy theories)? For some people, situational attributions are scary! The possibility of life going wrong suddenly all by itself without humanity as the cause, or as Solomon stated, "Time and chance happen to us all", is frightening! It is much less alarming to believe in dispositional attributions where a person(s) is at fault for what happened. Think about it. If life went wrong on its own, that's scary because I don't have any control over that. But if life went wrong because of a person, I have some control by preventing that person from ever causing chaos again.

---

**Related Verses:**
*Isaiah 43:2, Proverbs 3:5-6, II Timothy 1:7*

# DAILY M.E.D.S.:
*Apply this tool to receive the medicinal benefits of the devotional from the previous page.*

### MEDITATE:
Reflect upon the content of this devotional. Write, recite and mull over the key verses repeatedly until they reach your heart.

_____
_____
_____
_____

### ENGAGE:
Discuss this devotional with a trusted spiritual friend, pastor or counselor. Share your struggles relating to this devotional. Write whatever significant feedback they offer you. Most importantly, incorporate this devotional into your prayer life.

_____
_____
_____
_____

### DECIDE:
Consider the practical decisions you must make regarding this devotional. Write down those decisions and seek someone to keep you accountable.

_____
_____
_____
_____

### SURVEY:
Take note of your progress regarding this devotional. Changes don't happen suddenly but subtly. Write down any subtle improvements you notice over some time.

_____
_____
_____
_____

# EXISTENTIAL THREATS

*"He that dwelleth in the secret place of the Most High shall abide under the shadow of the Almighty... under His wings you will find refuge." Psalm 91:1.*

I once probed a retired Science Professor from Brown University about his theories on God. "I started my profession as an atheist and came out as a believer on the backend. When I realized the dozens of existential threats we face, yet we remain on planet earth thousands of years later, I had to conclude that some Sovereign Hand must be protecting us." Nuclear war, bioengineered pandemics, nanotechnology, climate change, and cyberterrorism are just a few things that put us all at risk. The one common denominator between all existential threats is reckless people. Of course, a meteor could annihilate the planet. But it's more likely we implode from the doings of the dastardly than explode from a foreign agent. God promised He would never again destroy the earth by flood, but He didn't say we wouldn't.

Paranoia is not only psychosis but a typical human experience, at least in its milder form. An experiment in London revealed that 40% of mentally stable passengers on a virtual train ride assessed their computerized passengers as dangerous even though they were programmed to be emotionally neutral (Freeman, 2008). At least once in your life, you'll experience paranoia related to your fellow species. Some psychologists theorize that paranoia stems from earlier trauma whereby you experienced the darker side of humanity and merely expect it to happen again. In other words, you're not crazy, just logically anticipating what has already proven to be true. Some paranoia (minus the delusions) is the outcome of simply paying careful attention; an astute awareness of existential threats.

Inside the Holy of Holies, warring angels or militant cherubim hover the mercy seat with outstretched wings. When the psalmist mentions taking refuge "under His wings," he's alluding to these angels. God appoints cherubim to keep His people safe from all impending doom. Psalm 91 teaches us that making it a practice to abide in His presence heightens our awareness of these militant cherubim who wage war on our behalf. The remedy for paranoia is not pretending the world isn't dangerous but realizing God's angels are far more treacherous than any peril approaching your doorway.

---

### Related Verses:
*Psalm 91:11-12, Psalm 121:7-8, Joshua 1:9*

Dr. JESUS

# DAILY M.E.D.S.:
*Apply this tool to receive the medicinal benefits of the devotional from the previous page.*

## MEDITATE:
Reflect upon the content of this devotional. Write, recite and mull over the key verses repeatedly until they reach your heart.

_____
_____
_____
_____

## ENGAGE:
Discuss this devotional with a trusted spiritual friend, pastor or counselor. Share your struggles relating to this devotional. Write whatever significant feedback they offer you. Most importantly, incorporate this devotional into your prayer life.

_____
_____
_____
_____

## DECIDE:
Consider the practical decisions you must make regarding this devotional. Write down those decisions and seek someone to keep you accountable.

_____
_____
_____
_____

## SURVEY:
Take note of your progress regarding this devotional. Changes don't happen suddenly but subtly. Write down any subtle improvements you notice over some time.

_____
_____
_____
_____

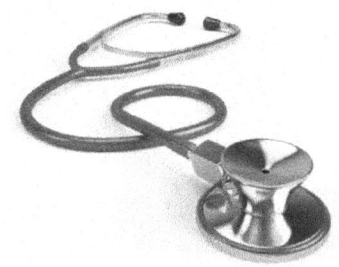

# POST-TRAUMATIC STRESS DISORDER:

*The stress resulting from the suffering or witnessing of a catastrophic event which includes abuse, abandonment, a serious accident, war, or sudden deaths of loved ones.*

RELEVANT BIBLICAL PERSONALITIES:
Job (Job 19:23-27)
Post-Flood Noah (Genesis 9:21)
Survivors of Babylon (Psalm 137)
Nehemiah's People (Nehemiah 4:14)
Demoniac Man (Matthew 8:28)

# P.T.S.D.

*"The wind ceased, and there was a great calm. Then, Jesus said to them, 'Why are you still afraid? Do you still have no faith?'" Mark 4:39*

Standing within proximity of a shotgun firing, you hear reverberation long after the detonation. The sound of humming or buzzing lasts for a while after the blast. Likewise, just because a crisis has ended in reality - an abusive relationship, a bloody battle, a sexual violation - doesn't mean it's concluded in mentality. The crisis persists long after you move out of his house, fly home from Iraq or watch your perpetrator escorted away in handcuffs. Just like the experience with the shotgun, the reverberation outlasts the detonation.

The Amygdala is an indispensable region of your brain that works like an alarm clock. It awakens you from a lackadaisical posture so that you can fittingly respond to an attacker bum-rushing you with a knife or some other imminent situation. Without your Amygdala, you'd die a fool's death in the prime of your life. Like Grandmaster Flash said, "It's a jungle sometimes, and I wonder how I'll be kept from going under." The Amygdala is an alarming sensation that keeps you alive in a capricious world. P.T.S.D. develops as a result of the Amygdala failing to shut off. The alarm clock won't stop blaring, and relaxation becomes impossible! When P.T.S.D. takes full measure, every circumstance feels like a crisis as you live within the constant reverberation of what was.

In our focal passage, the storm has ceased, yet the disciples remain frazzled. There was a calm in the air but no calmness between their ears. Jesus' question is not as much a rebuke as it appeals to their reason and faith. The Savior hopes to disengage their Amygdala while activating their Prefrontal Cortex (critical reasoning) with such a question. "Why are you still afraid?". In other words, think this through. You are not in danger. Instead, you're standing in the safety of my presence. An abiding faith in Christ substantiated by lucidity is the best weapon to combat a limbic system gone mad.

---

## Related Verses:
*Matthew 24:6-13, Philippians 4:6, Psalm 23:4*

# DAILY M.E.D.S.:

*Apply this tool to receive the medicinal benefits of the devotional from the previous page.*

### MEDITATE:
Reflect upon the content of this devotional. Write, recite and mull over the key verses repeatedly until they reach your heart.

_____
_____
_____
_____

### ENGAGE:
Discuss this devotional with a trusted spiritual friend, pastor or counselor. Share your struggles relating to this devotional. Write whatever significant feedback they offer you. Most importantly, incorporate this devotional into your prayer life.

_____
_____
_____
_____

### DECIDE:
Consider the practical decisions you must make regarding this devotional. Write down those decisions and seek someone to keep you accountable.

_____
_____
_____
_____

### SURVEY:
Take note of your progress regarding this devotional. Changes don't happen suddenly but subtly. Write down any subtle improvements you notice over some time.

_____
_____
_____
_____

# WHAT MAKES YOU FEEL SAFE?
*"He prepares a table before me in the presence of my enemies." Psalm 23*

Bolted doors, a 35mm under your pillow, and a house in the hills will NOT fully satiate your need for safety. Moving out of Boston or N.Y.C. into rural America won't make you feel as secure as you suppose. Instead, these security measures reinforce the fact that you live in a capricious world. Soon, you'll toss and turn throughout the night, wondering, "If I'm safe, then why do I need a gun?" The adage is true - you can run, but you can't hide. What will make me feel secure if safety cannot be found in a loaded weapon or a remote location?

Abraham Maslow (Maslow, 1943) theorized that you'd never manifest your potential until you feel safe. Maslow's model suggested that the need to feel safe is pivotal for success in all avenues of life. Since 1946, Maslow's theory has been demonstrated through countless studies where participants do better when they feel safe. Students perform better on tests, adults with addictions stay sober longer, and employees achieve higher benchmarks when they feel safe. Once again, if safety is so paramount, what will make me feel secure?

Oddly enough, in Psalm 23, the songwriter does not describe safety as the distance from danger. The psalmist doesn't say, "He prepares a table before me far from my enemies." Instead, he depicts the safe place as being close to whatever threatens - eg. "...in the presence of my enemies". The formula for safety is when the presence of God mightily presides wherever danger closely resides. You don't feel genuinely covered by an umbrella until the rains come down hard, you don't feel protected by an anchor until the waves are raging and you won't feel sheltered by God until the enemy's breathing down your neck.

---

### Related Verses:
*Psalm 4:8, Deuteronomy 31:6, Hebrews 13:5*

# DAILY M.E.D.S.:

*Apply this tool to receive the medicinal benefits of the devotional from the previous page.*

## MEDITATE:
Reflect upon the content of this devotional. Write, recite and mull over the key verses repeatedly until they reach your heart.

_____
_____
_____
_____

## ENGAGE:
Discuss this devotional with a trusted spiritual friend, pastor or counselor. Share your struggles relating to this devotional. Write whatever significant feedback they offer you. Most importantly, incorporate this devotional into your prayer life.

_____
_____
_____
_____

## DECIDE:
Consider the practical decisions you must make regarding this devotional. Write down those decisions and seek someone to keep you accountable.

_____
_____
_____
_____

## SURVEY:
Take note of your progress regarding this devotional. Changes don't happen suddenly but subtly. Write down any subtle improvements you notice over some time.

_____
_____
_____
_____

# REPAIRING THE DAMAGE OF CHILDHOOD SEXUAL ABUSE

*"Do you not know that your body is a temple of God...you are not your own!" I Corinthian 6:19*

More than 50% of the victims of Childhood Sexual Abuse (CSA) grow up to become targets of domestic violence. Furthermore, 31% of CSA victims are sexually assaulted again by a known or unknown perpetrator later in life (Crime Survey for England and Wales, 2016). Like wounded fish preyed upon by sharks, the emotionally fractured find themselves hunted again and again by human predators. Just as the smell of blood allures sharks, the scent of emotional vulnerability attracts human offenders.

'Damaged goods' is a theme that surfaces in the data from survivors of CSA in reference to how they perceive themselves. A sense of being morally corrupt, or unworthy, stem from the erroneous notion that "I should have stopped the abuse, but I didn't". Feelings of being perverted derive from the memory that "It felt good when I was abused"; the body often betrays the soul by being sensually stimulated by the abuse. Of course, this arousal is not a reflection of the victim's character but merely a physiological response to being touched in sensitive areas. When survivors misinterpret these experiences, they see themselves as trashy.

This insecure self-image manifests itself through a lack of boundaries. In fact, an etymology of the term, "Insecurity", speaks volumes - the prefix, "In" means "Without" whereas the suffix, "Security" connotes boundaries. I can always detect how emotionally secure a person is by how comfortably they enforce boundaries. Just as the etymology teaches us, an insecure person is someone who lacks security measures or is without boundaries. Let me break it down like this. You will find very little security measures surrounding a junk yard. Conversely, you will notice all kinds of security measures inside of a bank. Why? Because boundaries are only enforced where valuables are realized. Likewise, survivors of CSA often lack boundaries because they see themselves as a junkyard rather than a bank.

The power of God's promises featured in the bible is that they shift one's eyes from loathing self to the loving Savior. One such example is I Corinthians 6:19 which reminds us that we belong to the One who made us with His word and redeemed us with His blood. How does this bring healing to survivors of CSE? Through the lens of the bible, worth is not discovered in WHO you are but WHOSE you are. You belong to Him, and that's what makes you worth protecting. I remember reading a plaque on my wall that my aunt stitched for me every night before I fell asleep as a child, "I know I'm somebody special, because God don't make no junk".

---

**Related Verses:**
*Psalms 139:14, Galatians 3:13, Matthew 18:10-14, Luke 15:8-10*

Dr. JESUS

# DAILY M.E.D.S.:
*Apply this tool to receive the medicinal benefits of the devotional from the previous page.*

## MEDITATE:
Reflect upon the content of this devotional. Write, recite and mull over the key verses repeatedly until they reach your heart.

_____
_____
_____
_____

## ENGAGE:
Discuss this devotional with a trusted spiritual friend, pastor or counselor. Share your struggles relating to this devotional. Write whatever significant feedback they offer you. Most importantly, incorporate this devotional into your prayer life.

_____
_____
_____
_____

## DECIDE:
Consider the practical decisions you must make regarding this devotional. Write down those decisions and seek someone to keep you accountable.

_____
_____
_____
_____

## SURVEY:
Take note of your progress regarding this devotional. Changes don't happen suddenly but subtly. Write down any subtle improvements you notice over some time.

_____
_____
_____
_____

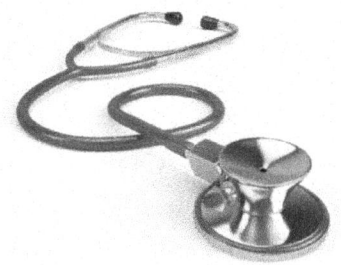

# RELATIONSHIP STRIFE:

*Inability to resolve conflicts and strife within relationships.*

<u>RELEVANT BIBLICAL PERSONALITIES:</u>
Paul & Barnabas (Act 15:36-41)
Jacob & Esau (Genesis 32)
Stranger in the crowd (Luke 12:13)
Prodigal's Older Brother (Luke 15:25-32)
Cain & Abel (Genesis 4)
Adam (Genesis 3:12)

## DOES IT MAKE SENSE TO LOVE HATERS?

*"Love your enemies and pray for those who persecute you s  
that you become sons/daughters of your Father in heaven." Matthew 5:44*

Careful analysis shows that the Christian ethic is the RIGHT thing to do and the BRIGHT thing to do. The gospel is not only moral but supremely intelligent, proving to be the wisest response to life's challenges. For instance, here are three reasons why the Christian ethic of loving your enemies is the savvy thing to do. Please understand that the Greek term for love (agape) refers to an intentional action to love someone, not necessarily like them.

1. Your MOTIONS influence your EMOTIONS. Researchers from Stanford University analyzed 19 million tweets regarding the Michael Brown shooting in Ferguson (Shashkevich, 2019). Researchers discovered that a hateful tweet was often followed by a more intense nasty tweet from the same individual, indicating that our actions amplify our emotions. How we act towards people influences how we feel about them. Therefore, if you want to stop hating your enemies, start as soon as possible with acts of love towards them.

2. Your attitude towards your haters will spill over into your attitude towards others. The notion that you can hate one person exclusively without it influencing how you feel about others is as ludicrous as believing that metastatic cancer will stay put in one organ. Displacement, a modern psychology theory, teaches us that we often misfire our hostile feelings at innocent targets. Therefore, if you care about your family and friends, start loving your foes. Or else your family and friends will eventually be affected by the hate towards your foes.

3. What you do determines who you become. Jesus states that we "become sons/daughters of God" by loving our enemies. Every action is a seed that grows into an attribute. We are all in the process of becoming lovers or haters.

---

### Related Verses:
*Romans 12:20, Genesis 45:4-6, Proverbs 25:21-22*

Dr. JESUS

# DAILY M.E.D.S.:
*Apply this tool to receive the medicinal benefits of the devotional from the previous page.*

## MEDITATE:
Reflect upon the content of this devotional. Write, recite and mull over the key verses repeatedly until they reach your heart.

_____
_____
_____
_____

## ENGAGE:
Discuss this devotional with a trusted spiritual friend, pastor or counselor. Share your struggles relating to this devotional. Write whatever significant feedback they offer you. Most importantly, incorporate this devotional into your prayer life.

_____
_____
_____
_____

## DECIDE:
Consider the practical decisions you must make regarding this devotional. Write down those decisions and seek someone to keep you accountable.

_____
_____
_____
_____

## SURVEY:
Take note of your progress regarding this devotional. Changes don't happen suddenly but subtly. Write down any subtle improvements you notice over some time.

_____
_____
_____
_____

## WHEN SHOULD I GIVE SOMEONE ANOTHER CHANCE?

*"Take Mark & bring him to me. For he is profitable to me within this ministry."*
*II Timothy 4:11.*

Back in the day, my favorite part of playing Atari was a mechanism known as the Reset-Button. The Reset-Button permitted me another chance to leap over rolling barrels while rescuing my duchess from Donkey Kong's captivity. Fortunately, there are Reset-Buttons within the Christian Journey that God presses for us ('His mercies are new every morning')....and we are expected to push those Reset-Buttons for others. But when do you press the Reset-Button for others who have failed you? When should you give someone another chance? Paul wisely discharged Mark from a missionary journey in earlier years because he deserted him on their voyage. In our verse, he gives Mark another chance but ONLY after two elements have come to fruition – TIME and SPACE.

First, there's TIME. In a systematic review of 200 studies on human behavior, researchers concluded that reducing personality flaws is possible, such as a choleric temperament mellowing out, but only after a process of time (Roberts, 2017). A big ship can turn in a different direction but not suddenly; instead, slowly and subtly. In the case of Mark, many years passed before Paul welcomed him back into the ministry; evidently, seasons whereby the momma's boy, Mark, matured into a reliable man. Time, sometimes, makes a mature man/woman out of the fools who wronged you.

Second, there's SPACE. The notion that you can accurately assess a person's character while cuddling in bed with them every night is as ludicrous as believing a fish can define water. Anytime you are immersed in a situation (such as the fish immersed in water), you lack the objectivity to determine what's happening clearly. For instance, many women believe that their batterer is Prince Charming while they remain in the relationship. But after they escape, they become astute to the nature of their oppressor. Paul took lots of space from Mark, and that space allowed him to spot noticeable changes. My kids know when I've gained weight, but only after seeing me return from some long trip. In summary, you need time & space from someone who wronged you before giving them another chance.

---

### Related Verses:
*Matthew 18:17, Genesis 13:8-9, Proverbs 4:23*

# DAILY M.E.D.S.:

*Apply this tool to receive the medicinal benefits of the devotional from the previous page.*

## MEDITATE:
Reflect upon the content of this devotional. Write, recite and mull over the key verses repeatedly until they reach your heart.

_____
_____
_____
_____

## ENGAGE:
Discuss this devotional with a trusted spiritual friend, pastor or counselor. Share your struggles relating to this devotional. Write whatever significant feedback they offer you. Most importantly, incorporate this devotional into your prayer life.

_____
_____
_____
_____

## DECIDE:
Consider the practical decisions you must make regarding this devotional. Write down those decisions and seek someone to keep you accountable.

_____
_____
_____
_____

## SURVEY:
Take note of your progress regarding this devotional. Changes don't happen suddenly but subtly. Write down any subtle improvements you notice over some time.

_____
_____
_____
_____

# ANNOYING PEOPLE

*"The FRUIT of the Spirit is love, joy, peace, patience, kindness, goodness, gentleness, faithfulness, and self-control." Galatians 5:22.*

Bugs don't just mess with your macaroni salad at the picnic but play a pivotal role in helping crops germinate. Strangely enough, without specific bugs in your garden, your tomatoes might wither away. Bugs aid in decomposing plant material and help pollinate the produce in your orchard. Bugs are more than just pests but needed organisms for crops to grow. In the same manner, consider the people in your life who "bug" you on the regular. You know, that lady who only shows up on your Facebook wall to find fault with something you post but never to support what you share. You know, that cousin who throws passive-aggressive digs about your unemployment or single status or whatever else. Thank God for "pests" who cultivate within you "fruit of the Spirit".

If you assume that virtues such as "patience" or "self-control" are fixed personality traits, you are mistaken! Brain mappings (sophisticated brain scans) reveal that our mind is malleable and forever in motion. So, how do we reshape our minds? Not just by reading the Word of God but applying it within our circumstances. According to a 2012 study (Schnitker, 2012), our responses to three areas of life help us grow in patience. The third area is daily hassles, such as getting stuck behind a school bus or anything that would inspire a snarky tweet. The second area is life's hardships. And the number one area where we grow in patience is, you guessed it, 'pests' - people who bug you with their annoying ways.

In our cancel culture, we quickly defriend all the people who get on our nerves (of course, some need to be blocked). It seems that we've done ourselves an excellent service by exterminating these pests. But if you pay attention to yourself over the next year or decade, you'll realize that your tolerance for any annoyance whatsoever is shrinking. Some call that shrinking tolerance "getting older." Rather than exterminating every pest, embrace them as opportunities to cultivate the character of Christ.

---

### Related Verses:
*Proverbs 27:17, Romans 5:4, I Corinthians 13:4-7*

# DAILY M.E.D.S.:

*Apply this tool to receive the medicinal benefits of the devotional from the previous page.*

## MEDITATE:
Reflect upon the content of this devotional. Write, recite and mull over the key verses repeatedly until they reach your heart.

_____
_____
_____
_____

## ENGAGE:
Discuss this devotional with a trusted spiritual friend, pastor or counselor. Share your struggles relating to this devotional. Write whatever significant feedback they offer you. Most importantly, incorporate this devotional into your prayer life.

_____
_____
_____
_____

## DECIDE:
Consider the practical decisions you must make regarding this devotional. Write down those decisions and seek someone to keep you accountable.

_____
_____
_____
_____

## SURVEY:
Take note of your progress regarding this devotional. Changes don't happen suddenly but subtly. Write down any subtle improvements you notice over some time.

_____
_____
_____
_____

# HOW DO YOU KNOW YOU'VE FORGIVEN?
*"Love your enemies, bless those who curse you, do good to those who hate you..."*
*Matthew 5:44*

How do you know that you've forgiven your offenders? I can profess to be smart all day long...But, if I don't measure up to the standards of intelligence on an IQ test, I'm just a blowhard. Criterions are established within every domain of life to determine whether we really possess what we profess. I've told my kids for years that I'm 5'7, but it wasn't until my Olivia took out the measuring tape the other day that she believed me (she actually said that I'm 5'8 with the hairdo - lolol). Anyway, here are a couple of measurements for forgiveness that align with the scriptures and the science.

Studies in behavioral science indicate two aspects of forgiveness - Decisional and Emotional. Decisional Forgiveness is the action to serve those who've offended you which aligns with Jesus' words in Matthew 5:44, "Do good to those who harm you." Examples of Decisional Forgiveness range from a letter of pardon to the folks who hurt you to something like Nelson Mandella's inaugural dinner invitation to the guard who urinated on him during his 27 years of wrongful imprisonment. Emotional Forgiveness involves feelings of empathy, sorrow and sometimes fondness towards the perpetrator. Emotional Forgiveness aligns with Jesus' words, "Bless those who curse you" (Matthew 5:44) the term bless implying a favorable posture of the heart towards someone. Decisional Forgiveness is an action whereas Emotional Forgiveness is an attitude.

Emotional Forgiveness seems the most elusive. How on earth do I manufacture empathy towards someone who urinated on me? The earlier research of William James (1890) showed that our bodily motions influence emotions; for instance, clenching your jaw escalates your frustration towards someone whereas serving them a cup of tea increases your fondness. The key to experiencing emotional forgiveness is decisional forgiveness. Do good towards someone, and you'll start to feel good about them (Caveat - you may never like them in an admirable sense of the word). As CS Lewis once stated, "Do not waste time bothering whether you 'love' someone; just act as if you do. As soon as you do this, you find one of the great secrets. When you are behaving as if you love someone, you will presently come to love them."

---

**Related Verses:**
*Matthew 5:7, Luke 23:34, Mark 11:25-26, Luke 11:4*

# DAILY M.E.D.S.:

*Apply this tool to receive the medicinal benefits of the devotional from the previous page.*

## MEDITATE:
Reflect upon the content of this devotional. Write, recite and mull over the key verses repeatedly until they reach your heart.

_____
_____
_____
_____

## ENGAGE:
Discuss this devotional with a trusted spiritual friend, pastor or counselor. Share your struggles relating to this devotional. Write whatever significant feedback they offer you. Most importantly, incorporate this devotional into your prayer life.

_____
_____
_____
_____

## DECIDE:
Consider the practical decisions you must make regarding this devotional. Write down those decisions and seek someone to keep you accountable.

_____
_____
_____
_____

## SURVEY:
Take note of your progress regarding this devotional. Changes don't happen suddenly but subtly. Write down any subtle improvements you notice over some time.

_____
_____
_____
_____

## HATED W/OUT JUST CAUSE

*"Then Amnon (after he raped his half-sister Tamar) hated her with intense hatred."*
II Samuel 13:15

Suppose you met Amnon at a party after he raped his sister, Tamar, and you inquired about her without knowledge of what happened. He'd probably vent about Tamar being a rotten person. He'd quite possibly dub her a jezebel and a narcissist. How many occasions have you listened to someone fume about their ex-spouse, or former employer, or whomever, being the spawn of satan? You walk away thinking, "That ex-spouse (or whomever) must be really terrible for such hatred to be directed towards them!". If that's your assumption, you need a lesson in human behavior 101. Surprisingly, hatred is often a coverup emotion for other things.

So, why does Amnon intensely hate Tamar? An experiment conducted by a behavioral scientist, Glass (1964), sheds some some light on this question. Glass conducted an experiment where participants negatively changed their view of other participants after shocking those subjects with an electrical device. Imagine! The culprits became disgusted with their victims after injuring them. Glass' experiment taught us that we judge the people we hurt as terrible in order to justify our actions against them as tolerable. The mind plays a trick on itself to protect itself from feelings of guilt. This also explains the white man's loathing of the black man after kidnapping him from his motherland and turning him into a slave. Amnon hates his sister, not because she hurt him, but because he hurt her. In short, we hate the ones we hurt.

So, next time you meet someone venting about someone they hate, don't be so quick to buy into the idea of that person being terrible. What lies beneath that hatred is not always evident at first glance. Behind that acrimony might be some awful act of betrayal or injustice the venter committed towards the one they loathe. Mark Twaine once stated, "There's the reason people give you. And then, there's the real reason."

---

**Related Verses:**
*Proverbs 18:17, Luke 12:14, Proverbs 10:18, Exodus 20:16*

# DAILY M.E.D.S.:
*Apply this tool to receive the medicinal benefits of the devotional from the previous page.*

## MEDITATE:
Reflect upon the content of this devotional. Write, recite and mull over the key verses repeatedly until they reach your heart.

_____
_____
_____
_____

## ENGAGE:
Discuss this devotional with a trusted spiritual friend, pastor or counselor. Share your struggles relating to this devotional. Write whatever significant feedback they offer you. Most importantly, incorporate this devotional into your prayer life.

_____
_____
_____
_____

## DECIDE:
Consider the practical decisions you must make regarding this devotional. Write down those decisions and seek someone to keep you accountable.

_____
_____
_____
_____

## SURVEY:
Take note of your progress regarding this devotional. Changes don't happen suddenly but subtly. Write down any subtle improvements you notice over some time.

_____
_____
_____
_____

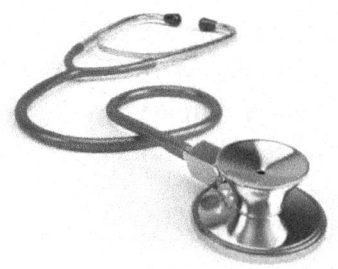

# STRESS:

*Feelings of being overwhelmed or unable to cope with mental or emotional pressure*

### RELEVANT BIBLICAL PERSONALITIES:
Paul (II Corinthians 4:9)

Jesus (Matthew 26:39)

Martha (Luke 10:40)

Moses (Numbers 11:10-15)

# IS HINDSIGHT 20/20?

*"Didn't we say to you in Egypt, 'Leave us alone; let us serve the Egyptians?'*
*It would have been better for us to serve the Egyptians than to die in the desert!"*
*Exodus 14:12.*

You've heard it said, "Hindsight is 20/20". Truth be told, "Hindsight is deceptive." Rosy Retrospection is a cognitive bias whereby you accentuate the positives of the past while dismissing its horrors (Side-note: 'dreary retrospection' is another cognitive bias that works the other way). Rosy Retrospection is so persuasive that a woman remembers her abuser as prince charming when she falls under this spell. Under this enchantment, yesterday is always better than today, and today won't be pleasurable until it becomes yesterday.

Rosy Retrospection happens for two reasons. First, it's a form of escapism from present stressful ordeals. The mind is notorious for seeking escape routes when under pressure; the past becomes a fantasy that allows the mind to relax from its immediate stress factors. Second, for some people, the traumas of the past are repressed. Repression is when you bury the pain of something so deeply that recollections become inaccessible. Within this repressed state of mind, only the positive sentiments of yesteryear float to the top.

Within our passage of study, the Jews fall under the spell of Rosy Retrospection. They look back at the sadistic Pharaoh and his vicious army with a smile. "Wasn't it so much better then!" they bellyache to sober-minded Moses, who endeavors to pave a better future. A little contextual analysis of the Jew's circumstances in this passage would prove my two reasons above to be right – they were under severe stress of not eating, and they had severe emotional pain probably repressed from the years in captivity. All this to say, if you find yourself obsessing about how wonderful it was back then, you better ask somebody! Your eyes are not to be trusted when glancing through a lens hazed with white light.

---

## Related Verses:
*Ecclesiastes 7:10, I Corinthians 10:13, Genesis 19:26*

Dr. JESUS

# DAILY M.E.D.S.:
*Apply this tool to receive the medicinal benefits of the devotional from the previous page.*

## MEDITATE:
Reflect upon the content of this devotional. Write, recite and mull over the key verses repeatedly until they reach your heart.

_____
_____
_____
_____

## ENGAGE:
Discuss this devotional with a trusted spiritual friend, pastor or counselor. Share your struggles relating to this devotional. Write whatever significant feedback they offer you. Most importantly, incorporate this devotional into your prayer life.

_____
_____
_____
_____

## DECIDE:
Consider the practical decisions you must make regarding this devotional. Write down those decisions and seek someone to keep you accountable.

_____
_____
_____
_____

## SURVEY:
Take note of your progress regarding this devotional. Changes don't happen suddenly but subtly. Write down any subtle improvements you notice over some time.

_____
_____
_____
_____

# FINANCIAL STRESS

*"I was glad when they said, "Let's go to the house of God." Psalm 122:1*

In a nation where 63% of constituents live paycheck to paycheck, keeping the wolf from the door is an everyday phenomenon. The Mind Over Money survey in 2020 reported that 77% of Americans worry about finances regularly. The happiest occasions – the birth of your child, a family wedding, or even a sunny day lounging at the beach - can be tainted by the angst of an impending bill. Financial stress is like a diseased fly that sits at the bottom of a precious ointment jar, spoiling its content. We are often too stressed (over money and other matters) to feel blessed. It's hard to loosen up when the wolf pounds on your door.

Good news! Research indicates that attending CHURCH buffers financial stress significantly more than other social activities (Krause, 2006). When researchers compared the psychological effects of the church with secular networks, they discovered that there is something relatively unique about being in the atmosphere of Worship. First, biblical teachings detach our souls from materialism while bringing us in line with heaven's value system. The church reminds us that relationships and personal growth are what matters the most. In the House of God, we are reminded that what truly counts cannot be counted. More importantly, we encounter Jehovah Jireh, the God who provides. The underlying thought process that fuels financial stress is that we are in this thing called life alone. Without the church, we exist as if we have to make our own way. The church reminds us that the Father in heaven who nurtures the birds of the air and dresses the lilies of the field underwrites our finances.

On a personal note, Sundays are the most restful for me. I'm usually delivering or listening to a message about how my benevolent Father meets all my needs. Before I hit the hay, I typically look up at the God whom I encountered earlier that morning in church and say, "Since you're awake all night, you figure this out. I'm going to sleep since there's no point in two of us being awake."

---

**Related Verses:**
*Philippians 4:19, Matthew 6:25-34, Psalm 107:7*

# DAILY M.E.D.S.:

*Apply this tool to receive the medicinal benefits of the devotional from the previous page.*

## MEDITATE:
Reflect upon the content of this devotional. Write, recite and mull over the key verses repeatedly until they reach your heart.

_____
_____
_____
_____

## ENGAGE:
Discuss this devotional with a trusted spiritual friend, pastor or counselor. Share your struggles relating to this devotional. Write whatever significant feedback they offer you. Most importantly, incorporate this devotional into your prayer life.

_____
_____
_____
_____

## DECIDE:
Consider the practical decisions you must make regarding this devotional. Write down those decisions and seek someone to keep you accountable.

_____
_____
_____
_____

## SURVEY:
Take note of your progress regarding this devotional. Changes don't happen suddenly but subtly. Write down any subtle improvements you notice over some time.

_____
_____
_____
_____

# BUSYNESS & STRESS

*"After the festival was over, while his parents were returning home, the boy Jesus stayed behind in Jerusalem, but they were unaware of it. Thinking he was in their company, they traveled on for a day." Luke 2:43-44.*

It is a strenuous mistake to confuse being ACTIVE with being PRODUCTIVE. Learn a hard lesson from the chickens. Our feathery friends expend more energy on the farm than any other animal. Hyper chickens will make an A.D.H.D. child seem like a poised monk meditating at the lakeside. Albeit chickens are active, they aren't nearly as productive as other sluggish animals. Maybe a few eggs are laid by the end of the day, even with their bobbling heads, fidgety feet, and twitchy wings. Whoopie-Do! All of their activity is not to be confused with productivity.

Furthermore, busyness and stress often go hand in hand. According to a study conducted by Farrand Ford in 1990, stress compromises the creative brain. Farrand Ford shows that stress results in well-rehearsed behavior patterns and automatic responses to the world around us. Stress squelches the spark of a novel idea, innovative solution, or creative thought. Busy, high-strung people get stuck in a high-speed yet monotonous replay of what happened yesterday, over and over again, every day. This science makes it clear that, like the chickens, you can be exceedingly active while being mildly productive.

In our passage of study, Joseph and Mary are on their way back home from the Passover festival. If you know anything about traveling on the animal in the ancient east, it was an involved endeavor that probably had their heads spinning. Prepare the animals, get the kids ready, install the proper straps, etc. So, here they are, busybodies heading back home from the feast. Only one problem – Joseph and Mary were so busy with their travels that they left Jesus behind! This unfortunate event is the outcome of busy, high-strung people. Losing touch with Jesus equates to severing your soul from the vine. Within this frame of mind, all creative juices stop flowing. All spiritual inclinations come to a halt. Apart from His presence, you can do nothing.

---

### Related Verses:
*John 15:4-11, Philippians 4:6, Proverbs 21:5*

# DAILY M.E.D.S.:

*Apply this tool to receive the medicinal benefits of the devotional from the previous page.*

## MEDITATE:
Reflect upon the content of this devotional. Write, recite and mull over the key verses repeatedly until they reach your heart.

_____
_____
_____
_____

## ENGAGE:
Discuss this devotional with a trusted spiritual friend, pastor or counselor. Share your struggles relating to this devotional. Write whatever significant feedback they offer you. Most importantly, incorporate this devotional into your prayer life.

_____
_____
_____
_____

## DECIDE:
Consider the practical decisions you must make regarding this devotional. Write down those decisions and seek someone to keep you accountable.

_____
_____
_____
_____

## SURVEY:
Take note of your progress regarding this devotional. Changes don't happen suddenly but subtly. Write down any subtle improvements you notice over some time.

_____
_____
_____
_____

# UNCERTAINTY & STRESS

*"I know the plans I have for you", declares the Lord. "Plans to prosper you and not to harm you." Jeremiah 29:11.*

A medical research team at U.C.L. conducted an experiment that compared the stress caused by physical agony with the stress of emotional uncertainty (Feller, 2016). Forty-five participants engaged in a computerized game while researchers measured their cortisol levels (stress hormone). The game's object was to determine the rocks where snakes were hiding; every time they turned over a rock with a snake, they received an electrical shock. The results indicated that cortisol levels were the highest, NOT when physical pain was the strongest, but when emotional uncertainty was the greatest; the moments when participants were the most unsure about where the snakes were hiding. The bottom line - Emotional uncertainty is far more stressful than physical agony.

Have you ever asked yourself, "Why do I keep going back to an abusive relationship? Why do I keep returning to harmful places?". Like a dog returning to its vomit, I keep revisiting toxic people, places, and things. One of the reasons you keep returning to painful places is because of its familiar scent. You know exactly what to expect in that abusive relationship. Even if it's painful, at least it's predictable!

Conversely, life outside your norms is scary as hell because you don't know what to anticipate. So, you go back to the devil you know, because it's better than the devil you don't know. Just as the U.C.L. researchers concluded, you would rather tolerate agony than deal with uncertainty.

In Jeremiah 29:11, when speaking about our future, God doesn't just promise to bless us, but He also pledges "not to harm" us. Why is that article included in this verse? For many of us with traumatic backgrounds, we dread looking out at what's ahead. We anticipate bad things happening to us when we step outside our comfort zone. For those of you petrified of moving forward, in the words of C.S. Lewis, "There are far better things ahead of us than anything we leave behind."

---

### Related Verses:
*Proverbs 3:5-6, Revelation 22:13, Romans 8:28*

Dr. JESUS

# DAILY M.E.D.S.:

*Apply this tool to receive the medicinal benefits of the devotional from the previous page.*

### MEDITATE:
Reflect upon the content of this devotional. Write, recite and mull over the key verses repeatedly until they reach your heart.

_____
_____
_____
_____

### ENGAGE:
Discuss this devotional with a trusted spiritual friend, pastor or counselor. Share your struggles relating to this devotional. Write whatever significant feedback they offer you. Most importantly, incorporate this devotional into your prayer life.

_____
_____
_____
_____

### DECIDE:
Consider the practical decisions you must make regarding this devotional. Write down those decisions and seek someone to keep you accountable.

_____
_____
_____
_____

### SURVEY:
Take note of your progress regarding this devotional. Changes don't happen suddenly but subtly. Write down any subtle improvements you notice over some time.

_____
_____
_____

# REFERENCES

Ariga, A. & Lleras, A. (2011). Brief and rare mental "breaks" keep you focused: Deactivation and reactivation of task goals preempt vigilance decrements. *Cognition*, March, 118(3).

Bouchard, T. (1979). The Minnesota Study of Twins Reared Apart. Retrieved from https://embryo.asu.edu/pages/sources-human-psychological-differences-minnesota-study-twins-reared-apart-1990-thomas-j

Bradshaw, M. et al. (2015). Listening to Religious Music and Mental Health in Later Life. *The Gerontologist*, 55(6), 961–971,

Buckingham, S. et al. (2013). Group Membership and Social Identity in Addiction Recovery. *Psychology of Addictive Behaviors*, 27(4).

Cherry, E. (1953). Some Experiments on the Recognition of Speech with One and Two Ears. *The Journal of the Acoustical Society of America*, 25, 975.

Cherry, K. (2020). Psychological Crisis Types and Causes. Retrieved from https://www.verywellmind.com/what-is-a-crisis-2795061

Cheung, Elaine & Gardner, Wendi. (2015). The Way I Make You Feel: Social Exclusion Enhances the Ability to Manage Others' Emotions. *Journal of Experimental Social Psychology*. 60(10).

Darley, J. M., & Latane, B. (1968). Bystander intervention in emergencies: Diffusion of responsibility. *Journal of Personality and Social Psychology*, 8(4), 377–383.

Day, Martin & Bobocel, D. (2013). The Weight of a Guilty Conscience: Subjective Body Weight as an Embodiment of Guilt. PloS one. 8. e69546. 10.1371/journal.pone.0069546

Deangelis, T. (2004). Consumerism and its Discontents. Retrieved from https://www.apa.org/monitor/jun04/discontents.

Feller, S (2016). Uncertainty causes more stress than inevitable pain. Retrieved from https://www.upi.com/Health_News/2016/03/29/Study-Uncertainty-causes-more-stress-than-inevitable-pain/1931459263700/.

Festinger, L. et al. (1963). Social Pressures in Informal Groups. Stanford: Stanford University Press.

Fitzsimmons-Craft E. E. (2017). Eating disorder-related social comparison in college women's everyday lives. *The International journal of eating disorders*, 50(8), 893-905.

Freeman D. (2008). Studying and treating schizophrenia using virtual reality: a new paradigm. *Schizophrenia*. 34(4):605-10

Gorka, S. et al. (2016). Intolerance of uncertainty and insula activation during uncertain reward. Cognitive, Affective, & Behavioral Neuroscience, 16, 929-939.

Locke, E. A. (1996). Motivation through conscious goal setting. *Applied & Preventive Psychology*, 5(2), 117-124.

Hibar, D. et al (2017). "Researchers create roadmap of bipolar disorder and how it affects the brain" (2017). Retrieved from https://news.usc.edu/120776/researchers-create-roadmap-of-bipolar-disorder-and-how-it-affects-the-brain

Kahneman, D. (1991). Anomalies: The Endowment Effect, Loss Aversion, and Status Quo Bias. *Journal of Economic Perspectives*, 5 (1): 193-206.

Kowalchyk, M. (2020). Narcissism through the lens of performative self-elevation. *Personality and Individual Differences*, 177.

Krause N. (2006). Gratitude Toward God, Stress, and Health in Late Life. *Research on Aging*. 28(2):163-183.

Kverme, B. (2019). Moving toward connectedness—A qualitative study of recovery processes for people with borderline personality disorder. *Frontiers in Psychology*, 10 (430).

Leary, M. (2004). The Psychology of Intellectual Humility. Retrieved from https://www.templeton.org/wp-content/uploads/2018/11/Intellectual-Humility-Leary-FullLength-Final.pdf

Levav, J. (2011). In Brief. Retrieved from https://www.apa.org/monitor/2011/06/inbrief.

Maslow, A. H. (1943). A theory of human motivation. *Psychological Review, 50*(4), 370–396.
Mauss, I. et al. (2011). Can Seeking Happiness Make People Happy? Paradoxical Effects of Valuing Happiness. *Emotion,* 11(4), 807-815.

Michel, A. (2016). Burnout and the brain. Retrieved from https://www.psychologicalscience.org/observer/burnout-and-the-brain.

Milgram, Stanley (1963). Behavioral Study of Obedience. *Journal of Abnormal and Social Psychology.* 67 (4): 371-8.

Miller G.A. et al. (1960). Plans and the Structure of Behavior. New York, NY: Henry Holt.

Oumaya M et al. (2008). Borderline personality disorder, self-mutilation and suicide: literature review. Encephale. Oct; 34(5), 452-8.

Park, B., & Rothbart, M. (1982). Perception of out-group homogeneity and levels of social categorization: Memory for the subordinate attributes of in-group and out-group members. *Journal of Personality and Social Psychology,* 42(6), 1051–1068.

Pereira, M. L. et al. (2015). Family functioning in adolescents with major depressive disorder: A comparative study. *Estudos de Psicologia, 32*(4), 641–652.

Petsko, E. (2018). The Surprising Link Between Language and Depression. Retrieved from https://www.mentalfloss.com/article/540559/surprising-link-between-language-and-depression.

Roberts, BW (2017). A systematic review of personality trait change through intervention. *Psychological Bulletin.* 143(2):117-141.

Roper, S et al. (1976). The spontaneous decay of compulsive urges. *Behaviour Research and Therapy,* 14(6), 445-453.

Schnitker, S. (2012). An examination of patience and well-being. *The Journal of Positive Psychology.* 7, 263-280.

Shashkevich, A. (2019). How people want to feel determines whether others can influence their emotions. Retrieved from https://news.stanford.edu/2019/06/13/examining-peoples-emotions-influenced-others/

Sheldon, K. M., Ryan, R., & Reis, H. T. (1996). What makes for a good day? Competence and autonomy in the day and in the person. *Personality and Social Psychology Bulletin, 22*(12), 1270-1279.

Sinha, Rajita. (2008). Chronic Stress, Drug use, and vulnerability to addiction. *Annals of New York Academy of Sciences,* October, P.105-130.

Straus, J. (2015). Sour Mood Getting You Down? Go Back to Nature. Retrieved from https://www.health.harvard.edu/mind-and-mood/sour-mood-getting-you-down-get-back-to-nature.

Weaver KE et al. (2013). Rural-urban differences in health behaviors and implications for health status among US cancer survivors. *Cancer Causes Control,* 24(8):1481-90.

Wilson, T. et al. (2014). Just Think: the challenges of the disengaged mind. *Sciencemag.org,* Volume 345, Issue 6192.

Wong et al. (2016). Does gratitude writing improve the mental health of psychotherapy clients? Evidence from a randomized controlled trial. *Psychotherapy Research, 28*(2).

Word, C. O. (1974). The nonverbal mediation of self-fulfilling prophecies in interracial interaction. *Journal of Experimental Social Psychology, 10*(2), 109–120.